ABC OF HEART FAILURE

Second Edition

ABC OF HEART FAILURE

Second Edition

Edited by

RUSSELL C DAVIS
Consultant Cardiologist and Senior Lecturer
University Department of Medicine, City Hospital, Birmingham

MICHAEL K DAVIES
Consultant Cardiologist and Senior Lecturer
Department of Cardiology, University Hospital Birmingham NHS Foundation Trust,
Queen Elizabeth Hospital, Birmingham

GREGORY Y H LIP
Consultant Cardiologist and Professor of Cardiovascular Medicine
University Department of Medicine, City Hospital, Birmingham

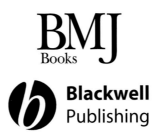

BMJ Books

Blackwell Publishing

© Blackwell Publishing Ltd 2006
BMJ Books is an imprint of the BMJ Publishing Group, used under licence

Blackwell Publishing Inc., 350 Main Street, Malden, Massachuesetts 02148–5020, USA
Blackwell Publishing Ltd, 9600 Garsington Road, Oxford OX4 2DQ, UK
Blackwell Publishing Asia Pty Ltd, 550 Swanston Street, Carlton, Victoria 3053, Australia

First published 2000
Second edition 2006

1 2006

Library of Congress Cataloging-in-Publication Data
Davis, Russell C., 1965–
ABC of heart failure / Russell C. Davis, Michael K. Davies, Gregory Y.H. Lip. — 2nd ed.
      p. ; cm.
    Previous ed. edited by Christopher R. Gibbs, Michael K. Davies, and Gregory Y.H. Lip.
    Includes bibliographical references and index.
    ISBN-13: 978-0-7279-1644-0
    ISBN-10: 0-7279-1644-0
  1. Heart failure. I. Davies, Michael K. II. Lip, Gregory Y. H. III. ABC of heart failure. IV. Title.
    [DNLM: 1. Heart Failure, Congestive. WG 370 D263a 2007]
  RC685.C53D38 2007
  616.1′29—dc22

                                      2006018527

ISBN-13: 978-0-7279-1644-0
ISBN-10: 0-7279-1644-0

A catalogue record for this book is available from the British Library

Cover image of conceptual computer artwork representing a heart attack is courtesy of David Mack/Science Photo Library

Set in 9/11 pts New Baskerville by Newgen Imaging System Pvt., Ltd, Chennai, India
Printed and bound in Singapore by Fabulous Printers Pte Ltd

Commissioning Editor: Eleanor Lines
Editorial Assistant: Vicky Pittman
Development Editor: Sally Carter / Vicki Donald
Production Controller: Debbie Wyer

For further information on Blackwell Publishing, visit our website:
www.blackwellpublishing.com

The publisher's policy is to use permanent paper from mills that operate a sustainable forestry policy, and which has been manufactured from pulp processed using acid-free and elementary chlorine-free practices. Furthermore, the publisher ensures that the text paper and cover board used have met acceptable environmental accreditation standards.

Blackwell Publishing makes no representation, express or implied, that the drug dosages in this book are correct. Readers must therefore always check that any product mentioned in this publication is used in accordance with the prescribing information prepared by the manufacturers. The author and the publishers do not accept responsibility or legal liability for any errors in the text or for the misuse or misapplication of material in this book.

Contents

Preface

Heart failure continues as a major healthcare problem due to its high prevalence rate and high mortality. Over recent years resources, facilities, and services for the diagnosis and treatment of heart failure patients have expanded substantially, and there have been major advances in pharmacological and device therapies available for treatment. In the light of these advances and developments, it is an appropriate time to update the *ABC of heart failure*, which aims to bring together practical information covering the spectrum of heart failure from epidemiology and diagnosis through to treatment and services. This second edition also brings up to date the information from which recent guidelines in Britain, Europe, and the United States have been based. The aim of this publication is not only to form a useful reference book but also to be a concise handbook for all those participating in the multidisciplinary teams looking after patients with heart failure. We wish to gratefully acknowledge the original contributions to the first edition by Professor D G Beevers, Dr C R Gibbs, Professor F D R Hobbs, Dr G Jackson, Dr T Millane, and Dr R D S Watson. Their original chapters have formed the basis for several of those in this expanded second edition. Dr Gibbs' contribution to the editing process of the first edition was especially valuable.

Russell C Davis
Michael K Davies
Gregory Y H Lip
Birmingham, UK

1 History and epidemiology

"The very essence of cardiovascular practice is the early detection of heart failure"
Sir Thomas Lewis, 1933

Heart failure is the end stage of most diseases of the heart and is a major cause of morbidity and mortality. It is estimated to account for about 5% of admissions to hospital medical wards, with over 100 000 annual admissions in the UK.

The overall prevalence of heart failure in the West Midlands region of England in the late 1990s, using objective criteria for diagnosis, was at least 2.3% in those aged ≥45, with a marked increase in prevalence with advancing age. The annual incidence of heart failure is 1–3 per 1000, and the relative incidence doubles for each decade of life after the age of 45. The overall prevalence is likely to increase in the future because of an ageing population and therapeutic advances in the management of acute myocardial infarction and established heart failure leading to improved survival in patients with impaired cardiac function.

Unfortunately, heart failure can be difficult to diagnose clinically as many features of the condition are not organ specific and there may be few clinical features in the early stages of the disease. Recent advances have made the early recognition of heart failure increasingly important as modern drug treatment has the potential to improve symptoms and quality of life, reduce rates of admission to hospital, slow the rate of disease progression, and improve survival. In addition, coronary revascularisation and heart valve surgery are now regularly performed, even in elderly patients.

A brief history

Descriptions of heart failure exist from ancient Egypt, Greece, and India, and the Romans were known to use the foxglove as medicine. Little understanding of the nature of the condition can have existed until William Harvey described the circulation in 1628. Röntgen's discovery of x rays and Einthoven's development of electrocardiography in the 1890s led to improvements in the investigation of heart failure. The development of echocardiography, cardiac catheterisation, and nuclear medicine has since improved the diagnosis and investigation of patients with heart failure. Blood letting and leeches were used as treatment for centuries, and William Withering published his account of the benefits of digitalis in 1785.

Some definitions of heart failure

- A condition in which the heart fails to discharge its contents adequately (Thomas Lewis, 1933)
- A state in which the heart fails to maintain an adequate circulation for the needs of the body despite a satisfactory filling pressure (Paul Wood, 1950)
- A pathophysiological state in which an abnormality of cardiac function is responsible for the failure of the heart to pump blood at a rate commensurate with the requirements of the metabolising tissues (E Braunwald, 1980)
- Heart failure is the state of any heart disease in which, despite adequate ventricular filling, the heart's output is decreased or in which the heart is unable to pump blood at a rate adequate for satisfying the requirements of the tissues with function parameters remaining within normal limits (H Denolin, H Kuhn, H P Krayenbuehl, F Loogen, A Reale, 1983)
- A clinical syndrome caused by an abnormality of the heart and recognised by a characteristic pattern of haemodynamic, renal, neural, and hormonal responses (Philip Poole-Wilson, 1985)
- [A] syndrome . . . which arises when the heart is chronically unable to maintain an appropriate blood pressure without support (Peter Harris, 1987)
- A syndrome in which cardiac dysfunction is associated with reduced exercise tolerance, a high incidence of ventricular arrhythmias, and shortened life expectancy (Jay Cohn, 1988)
- Abnormal function of the heart causing a limitation of exercise capacity or "ventricular dysfunction with symptoms (anonymous and pragmatic)
- Symptoms of heart failure, objective evidence of cardiac dysfunction, and response to treatment directed towards heart failure (Task Force of the European Society of Cardiology, 1995)

Adapted from Poole-Wilson PA, et al, eds, *Heart failure* New York: Churchill Livingstone, 1997:270)

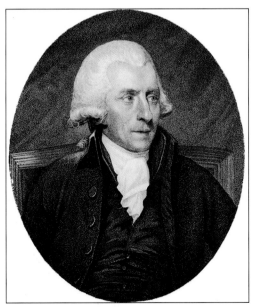

In 1785 William Withering of Birmingham published an account of the medicinal use of digitalis. Reproduced with permission from the Fine Arts Photographic Library

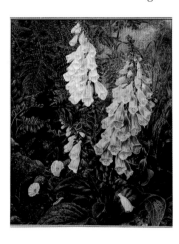

The foxglove was used as a medicine in heart disease as long ago as Roman times. Reproduced with permission from the Fine Arts Photographic Library

In the 19th and early 20th centuries, heart failure associated with fluid retention was treated with Southey's tubes, which were inserted into oedematous peripheries, allowing some drainage of fluid.

It was not until the 20th century that diuretics were developed. The early, mercurial agents, however, were associated with substantial toxicity, unlike the thiazide diuretics, which were introduced in the 1950s. Vasodilators were not widely used until the development of angiotensin converting enzyme inhibitors in the 1970s. The landmark CONSENSUS-I study (first cooperative north Scandinavian enalapril survival study), published in 1987, showed the unequivocal survival benefits of enalapril in patients with severe heart failure. The benefits of β blockers were established in the 1990s, and subsequently aldosterone antagonists and device therapy (resynchronisation therapy and implantable defibrillators) are becoming established treatments.

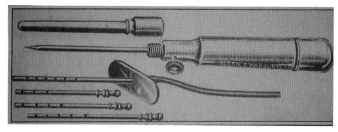

Southey's tubes were at one time used for removing fluid from oedematous patients

Epidemiology

Studies of the epidemiology of heart failure have been complicated by the lack of universal agreement on a definition of heart failure, which is primarily a clinical diagnosis. National and international comparisons have therefore been difficult, and mortality data, postmortem studies, and hospital admission rates are not easily translated into incidence and prevalence. Several different systems have been used in large population studies, with the use of scores for clinical features determined from history and examination, and, in most cases, chest radiography to define heart failure.

The Task Force on Heart Failure of the European Society of Cardiology has published guidelines on the diagnosis of heart failure, which require the presence of symptoms and objective evidence of cardiac dysfunction. Reversibility of symptoms on appropriate treatment is also desirable. Echocardiography is recommended as the best way of assessing cardiac function, and this investigation has been used in more recent studies.

In the Framingham heart study a cohort of 5209 participants has been assessed biennially since 1948, with a further cohort (their offspring) added in 1971. This uniquely large dataset has been used to determine the incidence and prevalence of heart failure, defined with consistent clinical and radiographic criteria.

Several UK studies of the epidemiology of heart failure and left ventricular dysfunction have been conducted, including a study of the incidence of heart failure in one west London district (Hillingdon heart failure study) and large prevalence studies in Glasgow (north Glasgow monitoring trends and determinants in cardiovascular disease (MONICA) study) and the West Midlands ECHOES (echocardiographic heart of England screening) study. Epidemiological studies of heart failure have used different levels of ejection fraction to define systolic dysfunction. The Glasgow study, for example, used an ejection fraction of 30% as its criterion, whereas most others have used levels of 40–45%. The prevalence of heart failure seems similar in many different surveys, however, despite variation in the levels of ejection fraction, and this observation is not entirely explained.

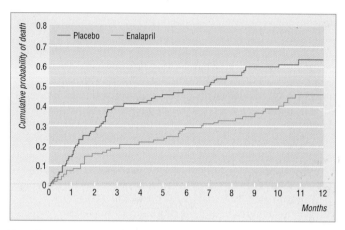

Mortality curves from the CONSENSUS-I study

European Society of Cardiology criteria for diagnosis of heart failure

- To satisfy the diagnosis of heart failure there must be:
  Appropriate symptoms
  Objective evidence of cardiac dysfunction
  and (in cases of doubt)
  Appropriate response to relevant treatment
- Echocardiography is the most practical tool to demonstrate cardiac dysfunction

---

The Framingham heart study has been the most important longitudinal source of data on the epidemiology of heart failure

---

Methods of assessing prevalence of heart failure in published studies

- Clinical and radiographic assessment
- Echocardiography
- General practice monitoring
- Drug prescription data

Prevalence of heart failure

During the 1980s, the Framingham study reported the age adjusted overall prevalence of heart failure, with similar rates for men and women. Prevalence increased dramatically with increasing age, with an approximate doubling in the prevalence of heart failure with each decade of ageing.

The MONICA study is an international study conducted under the auspices of the World Health Organization to monitor trends in and determinants of mortality from cardiovascular disease

In Nottinghamshire, the prevalence of heart failure in 1994 was estimated from prescription data for loop diuretics and examination of the general practice notes of a sample of these patients to determine the number who fulfilled predetermined criteria for heart failure. The overall prevalence of heart failure was estimated as 1.0% to 1.6%, rising from 0.1% in those aged 30–39 to 4.2% at 70–79 years. This method, however, may exclude individuals with mild heart failure and include patients treated with diuretics who do not have heart failure.

In the ECHOES study left ventricular systolic dysfunction was diagnosed in 1.8% of the 3960 participants, but half had no symptoms. Definite heart failure was seen in 2.3% and was associated with an ejection fraction of <40% in 41% of patients, atrial fibrillation in 33%, and valve disease in 26%. In total, 3.1% patients aged ≥45 had definite or probable heart failure.

Incidence of heart failure

The Framingham data show an age adjusted annual incidence of heart failure of 0.14% in women and 0.23% in men. Survival in women is generally better than in men, leading to the same point prevalence. There is an approximate doubling in the incidence of heart failure with each decade of ageing, reaching 3% in those aged 85–94 years.

The recent Hillingdon study examined the incidence of heart failure, defined on the basis of clinical and radiographic findings, with echocardiography in a population in west London. The overall annual incidence was 0.08%, rising from 0.02% at age 45–55 to 1.2% at age ≥86. About 80% of these patients received the first diagnosis after acute hospital admission, with only 20% being identified in general practice and referred to a dedicated clinic.

The Glasgow group of the MONICA study and the ECHOES group have found that coronary artery disease is the most powerful risk factor for impaired left ventricular function, either alone or in combination with hypertension. In these studies, hypertension alone did not seem to contribute substantially to impairment of left ventricular systolic contraction, though the Framingham study did report a more substantial contribution from hypertension. This apparent difference between the studies may reflect improvements in the treatment of hypertension and the fact that some patients with hypertension, but without coronary artery disease, may develop heart failure as a result of diastolic dysfunction.

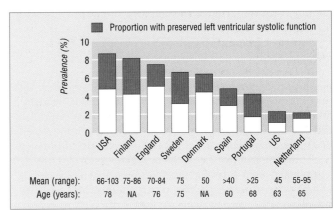

| Mean (range): | 66-103 | 75-86 | 70-84 | 75 | 50 | >40 | >25 | 45 | 55-95 |
| Age (years): | 78 | NA | 76 | 75 | NA | 60 | 68 | 63 | 65 |

Prevalence of heart failure in cross sectional population echocardiographic studies and proportion of patients with preserved left ventricular systolic function. Adapted from McMurray JJ, Pfeffer MA. *Lancet* 2005;365:1877–89)

Prevalence (percentage) of ejection fraction <40% and 40–50% by age and sex in the ECHOES study

	Male	**Female**	**Total**
Ejection fraction <40%			
Age (years):			
45–54	4/633 (0.6)	0/681	4/1314 (0.3)
55–64	19/623 (3.0)	3/571 (0.5)	22/1194 (1.8)
65–74	23/480 (4.8)	5/472 (1.1)	28/952 (2.9)
75–84	10/205 (4.9)	6/229 (2.6)	16/434 (3.7)
≥85	2/23 (8.7)	0/43	2/66 (3.0)
Total	58/1964 (3.0)	14/1996 (0.7)	72/3960 (1.8)
Ejection fraction 40–50%			
Age (years):			
45–54	8/633 (1.3)	9/681 (1.3)	17/1314 (1.3)
55–64	25/623 (4.0)	17/571 (3.0)	42/1194 (3.5)
65–74	32/480 (6.7)	13/472 (2.8)	45/952 (4.7)
75–84	13/205 (6.3)	13/229 (5.7)	26/434 (6.0)
≥85	3/23 (13.0)	6/43 (14.0)	9/66 (13.6)
Total	81/1964 (4.1)	58/1996 (2.9)	139/3960 (3.5)

Adapted from Davies MK, et al. *Lancet* 2001;358:439–44

Prevalence of left ventricular dysfunction

Large surveys were carried out in Britain in the 1990s, in Glasgow and the West Midlands, using echocardiography. In Glasgow the prevalence of significantly impaired left ventricular contraction in people aged 25–74 was 2.9%; in the West Midlands, the prevalence was 1.8% in those aged ≥45. The higher rates in the Scottish study may reflect the high prevalence of ischaemic heart disease, the main precursor of impaired left ventricular function in both studies. The numbers of symptomatic and asymptomatic cases were about the same in both studies.

> About half of the patients with measurable left ventricular dysfunction in the Glasgow and West Midlands studies had no symptoms and therefore would be difficult to identify at this relatively early stage by clinical examination—underscoring the need for echocardiography

Ethnic differences

Ethnic differences in the incidence of and mortality from heart failure have also been reported. In the US, African-American men have been reported as having a 33% greater risk of being

> In the US mortality from heart failure at age <65 has been reported as being up to 2.5-fold higher in black patients than in white patients

admitted to hospital for heart failure than white men; the risk for black women was 50% greater.

A similar picture emerged in a survey of heart failure among acute medical admissions to a city centre teaching hospital in Birmingham. The commonest underlying aetiological factors were coronary heart disease in white patients, hypertension in black Afro-Caribbean patients, and coronary heart disease and diabetes in Indo-Asians. Some of these racial differences may be related to the higher prevalence of hypertension and diabetes in black people and coronary artery disease and diabetes mellitus in Indo-Asians.

At eight years' follow-up of admissions for acute heart failure to a city centre hospital serving a multiethnic population, the total mortality was 90.5% among Europeans and 87.0% among non-Europeans (log rank test, P = 0.0705). The non-European patients had significantly better survival at all time points until six years, after which the survival curves start to converge.

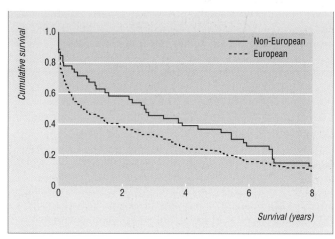

At 8 years' follow-up of acute heart failure admissions to a city centre hospital serving a multiethnic population, the total mortality was 90.5% amongst Europeans and 87.0% among non-Europeans (log rank test, P = 0.0705). The non-European patients had significantly better survival at all time points until 6 years, after which the survival curves start to converge. Sosin MD, et al. *Eur J Heart Fail* 2004;6:669–72

Summary of relative importance of aetiological factors by ethnic group based on available evidence

	White European	Black	South Asian
Ischaemic heart disease	+++	+	+++
Diabetes	++	+++	+++
Hypertension	++	+++	+
Atrial fibrillation	++	+	+
Dilated cardiomyopathy	+	++	No data
Increasing age	+++	++	++
Access to care	–	+	+

(+ = some importance, +++ = great importance)
Adapted from Sosin MD, et al. *Eur J Heart Fail* 2004:6:831–43

Impact on health services

Heart failure accounts for at least 5% of admissions to general medical and geriatric wards in British hospitals, and admission rates for heart failure in various European countries (Sweden, Netherlands, and Scotland) and in the US doubled between the 1980s and 1990s, although this increase has now levelled off. Furthermore, heart failure accounts for about 1.9% of the total healthcare expenditure in the UK, most of these costs being related to hospital admissions. The cost of heart failure is increasing, with an estimated UK expenditure in 2000 of £905m. "Indirect" costs (for example, on nursing home care) are equivalent to a further 2% of the NHS budget.

Hospital readmissions and general practice consultations often occur soon after the diagnosis of heart failure. In elderly patients with heart failure, readmission rates range from 29–47% within three to six months of the initial hospital discharge. Treating patients with heart failure with angiotensin converting enzyme inhibitors can reduce the overall cost of treatment (because of reduced hospital admissions), despite increased drug expenditure and improved long term survival.

Further reading

- Cowie MR, Wood DA, Coats AJS, Thompson SG, Poole-Wilson PA, Suresh V, et al. Incidence and aetiology of heart failure: a population-based study. *Eur Heart J* 1999;20:421–8.
- Davies MK, Hobbs FDR, Davis RC, Kenkre JE, Roalfe AK, Hare R, et al. Prevalence of left ventricular systolic dysfunction and heart failure in the echocardiographic heart of England screening study: a population based study. *Lancet* 2001;358:439–44.
- Ho KK, Pinsky JL, Kannel WB, Levy D. The epidemiology of heart failure: the Framingham study. *J Am Coll Cardiol* 1993;22:6–13A.
- McDonagh TA, Morrison CE, Lawrence A, Ford I, Tunstall-Pedoe H, McMurray JJV, et al. Symptomatic and asymptomatic left-ventricular systolic dysfunction in an urban population. *Lancet* 1997;350:829–33.
- Stewart S, Jenkins A, Buchan S, McGuire A, Capewell S, McMurray JJV. The current cost of heart failure to the National Health Service in the UK. *Eur J Heart Fail* 2002;4:361–71.
- Task Force on Heart Failure of the European Society of Cardiology. Guidelines for the diagnosis of heart failure. *Eur Heart J* 1995;16:741–51.

This chapter was adapted from the corresponding one in the first edition written by RC Davis, FDR Hobbs, and GYH Lip. Our colleague's previous contribution is gratefully acknowledged.

2 Aetiology

The relative importance of aetiological factors in heart failure depends on the population being studied as coronary artery disease and hypertension are common causes of heart failure in Western countries, whereas valvar heart disease and nutritional cardiac disease are more common in the developing world. Epidemiological studies also depend on the clinical criteria and relevant investigations used for diagnosis as it remains difficult, for example, to distinguish whether hypertension is the primary cause of heart failure or whether there is also underlying coronary artery disease.

Risk factors for coronary artery disease

Coronary heart disease is the commonest cause of heart failure in Western countries. In the studies of left ventricular dysfunction (SOLVD), coronary artery disease accounted for almost 75% of the cases of chronic heart failure in white men, though in the Framingham heart study, coronary heart disease accounted for only 46% of cases of heart failure in men and 27% of chronic heart failure cases in women. Coronary artery disease and hypertension (either alone or in combination) were implicated as the cause in over 90% of cases of heart failure in the Framingham study.

Recent studies that have allocated aetiology on the basis of non-invasive investigations—such as the Hillingdon heart failure study—have identified coronary artery disease as the primary cause in 36% of cases of heart failure. In the Hillingdon study, however, researchers could not identify the primary cause in 34% of cases. The related Bromley heart failure study used coronary angiography and myocardial perfusion scanning as well as historical and non-invasive findings to determine the aetiology of incident cases of heart failure. Coronary artery disease was the cause in at least 52%. As valve disease and atrial fibrillation were the cause in some of the remainder, coronary artery disease probably contributes to a substantially higher proportion of cases with left ventricular systolic dysfunction.

Coronary risk factors, such as smoking and diabetes mellitus, are also risk markers of the development of heart failure. Smoking is an independent and strong risk factor for the development of heart failure in men, though the findings in women are less consistent.

In the prevention arm of studies of left ventricular dysfunction, diabetes was an independent risk factor (about twofold) for mortality, the development of heart failure, and admission to hospital for heart failure, whereas in the Framingham study diabetes and left ventricular hypertrophy were the most significant risk markers of the development of heart failure. Body weight and a high ratio of total cholesterol to high density lipoprotein cholesterol concentration are also independent risk factors for heart failure. Clearly, these risk factors may increase the risks of heart failure through their effects on coronary artery disease, though diabetes alone may induce important structural and functional changes in the myocardium (sometimes known as "diabetic cardiomyopathy"), which further increase the risk of heart failure.

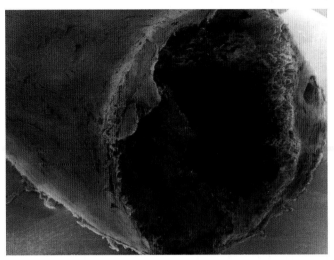

Blood clot in a coronary artery. With permission from the Science photo library/Professor PM Motta, G Macchiarelli, SA Nottola

---

Causes of heart failure

Coronary artery disease
- Myocardial infarction
- Ischaemia

Hypertension

Cardiomyopathy
- Dilated (congestive)
- Hypertrophic/obstructive
- Restrictive—for example, amyloidosis, sarcoidosis, haemochromatosis
- Obliterative

Diabetes mellitus

Valvar and congenital heart disease
- Mitral valve disease
- Aortic valve disease
- Atrial septal defect, ventricular septal defect

Arrhythmias
- Tachycardia
- Bradycardia (complete heart block, the sick sinus syndrome)
- Loss of atrial contraction—for example, atrial fibrillation

Alcohol and drugs
- Alcohol
- Cardiac depressant drugs (such as verapamil)
- Chemotherapeutic agents (such as doxorubicin)

"High output" failure
- Anaemia, thyrotoxicosis, arteriovenous fistulas, Paget's disease

Pericardial disease
- Constrictive pericarditis
- Pericardial effusion

Primary right heart failure
- Pulmonary hypertension—for example, pulmonary embolism, cor pulmonale

---

Effective lowering of blood pressure in patients with hypertension reduces the risk of heart failure; an overview of trials has estimated that effective antihypertensive treatment reduces the age standardised incidence of heart failure by up to 50%

Hypertension

Several epidemiological studies have shown that hypertension is associated with an increased risk of heart failure. In the Framingham heart study, hypertension was reported as the cause of heart failure—either alone or in association with other factors—in over 70% of cases, on the basis of non-invasive assessment. Other community and hospital based studies, however, have reported hypertension to be a less common cause of heart failure, and, indeed, the importance of hypertension as a cause of heart failure has been declining in the Framingham cohort since the 1950s. In the Bromley study of incident heart failure, hypertension was found to be the primary aetiology in only 4.4%, though 44% of patients had a history of hypertension. However, hypertension is probably a more common cause of heart failure in selected groups of patients, including women and black people.

Hypertension predisposes to the development of heart failure through several pathological mechanisms, including left ventricular hypertrophy. Left ventricular hypertrophy is associated with left ventricular systolic and diastolic dysfunction and an increased risk of myocardial infarction, and it predisposes to both atrial and ventricular arrhythmias. Electrocardiographic left ventricular hypertrophy is strongly correlated with the development of heart failure as it is associated with a 14-fold increase in the risk of heart failure in those aged ≤65 years. However, electrocardiography is still a relatively insensitive way of picking up left ventricular hypertrophy and may miss a considerable proportion of cases and echocardiography is a much more sensitive method.

Cardiomyopathies

Cardiomyopathies are diseases of heart muscle that are not secondary to coronary disease, hypertension, or congenital, valvar, or pericardial disease. As primary diseases of heart muscle, cardiomyopathies are less common causes of heart failure, but awareness of their existence is necessary to make a diagnosis. Cardiomyopathies are separated into four functional categories:

- dilated (congestive)
- hypertrophic
- restrictive, and
- obliterative.

These groups can include rare, specific diseases of the heart muscle (such as haemochromatosis (iron overload) and metabolic and endocrine disease), in which the heart is affected as part of a systemic disorder. Dilated cardiomyopathy is a more common cause of heart failure than hypertrophic and restrictive cardiomyopathies; obliterative cardiomyopathy is essentially limited to developing countries.

Dilated cardiomyopathy

Dilated cardiomyopathy describes disease of the heart muscle in which the predominant abnormality is dilatation of the left ventricle, with or without right ventricular dilatation. Myocardial cells are also hypertrophied, with increased variation in size and increased extracellular fibrosis. Family studies have reported that up to a quarter of cases of dilated cardiomyopathy have a familial basis (underscoring the need to offer echocardiographic screening to members of the patient's family). Viral myocarditis is a recognised cause; connective tissue diseases such as systemic lupus erythematosus, Churg-Strauss syndrome, and polyarteritis nodosa are rarer causes.

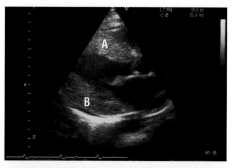

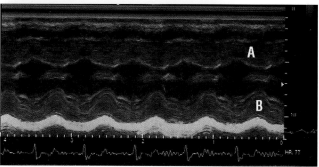

Two dimensional echocardiogram (top) and M mode echocardiogram (bottom) showing left ventricular hypertrophy. A = interventricular septum; B = ventricular wall

---

Causes of dilated cardiomyopathy

Familial

Infectious
- Viral (coxsackie B, cytomegalovirus, HIV)
- Rickettsia
- Bacteria (diphtheria)
- Mycobacteria
- Fungus
- Parasites (Chagas' disease, toxoplasmosis)
- Alcohol
- Cardiotoxic drugs (doxorubicin, zidovudine)
- Cocaine
- Iron overload (haemachromatosis and transfusional)
- Metals (cobalt, mercury, lead)
- Nutritional disease (beriberi, kwashiorkor, pellagra)
- Endocrine disease (myxoedema, thyrotoxicosis, acromegaly, phaeochromocytoma)

Pregnancy

Collagen disease
- Connective tissue diseases (systemic lupus erythematosus, scleroderma, polyarteritis nodosa)

Neuromuscular
- Duchenne's muscular dystrophy, myotonic dystrophy

Arrhythmias and heart failure: mechanisms

Tachycardias
- Reduce diastolic ventricular filling time
- Increase myocardial workload and myocardial oxygen demand, precipitating ischaemia
- If chronic, with poor rate control, they may lead to ventricular dilatation and impaired ventricular function ("tachycardia induced cardiomyopathy")

Bradycardias
- Compensatory increase in stroke volume is limited in the presence of structural heart disease, and cardiac output is reduced

Abnormal atrial and ventricular contraction
- Loss of atrial systole leads to the absence of active ventricular filling, which in turn lowers cardiac output and raises atrial pressure—for example, atrial fibrillation
- Dissociation of atrial and ventricular activity impairs diastolic ventricular filling, particularly in the presence of a tachycardia—for example, ventricular tachycardia

Idiopathic dilated cardiomyopathy is a diagnosis of exclusion. Coronary angiography will exclude coronary disease, and an endomyocardial biopsy is required to exclude underlying myocarditis or an infiltrative disease.

Dilatation can be associated with the development of atrial and ventricular arrhythmias, and dilatation of the ventricles leads to "functional" mitral and tricuspid valve regurgitation.

Hypertrophic cardiomyopathy

Hypertrophic cardiomyopathy has a strong familial inheritance (autosomal dominant), though sporadic cases may occur. It is characterised by abnormalities of the myocardial fibres, and in its classic form involves asymmetrical septal hypertrophy, which may be associated with aortic outflow obstruction (hypertrophic obstructive cardiomyopathy). Other forms also exist— apical hypertrophy (especially in Japan) and symmetrical left ventricular hypertrophy (where the echocardiographic distinction between this and hypertensive heart disease may be unclear). These abnormalities lead to poor left ventricular compliance, with high end diastolic pressures, and there is a common association with atrial and ventricular arrhythmias, the latter leading to sudden cardiac death. Mitral regurgitation may contribute to the development of heart failure in these patients, though many with hypertrophic cardiomyopathy do not have the full syndrome of heart failure.

Restrictive and obliterative cardiomyopathies

Restrictive cardiomyopathy is characterised by a stiff and poorly compliant ventricle, which is not substantially enlarged, and this is associated with abnormalities of diastolic function (relaxation) that limit ventricular filling. Systolic contraction is often preserved.

Amyloidosis and other infiltrative diseases, including sarcoidosis and haemochromatosis, can cause a restrictive syndrome. Endomyocardial fibrosis is also a cause of restrictive cardiomyopathy, though it is a rare cause of heart failure in Western countries. Endocardial fibrosis of the inflow tract of one or both ventricles, including the subvalvar regions, results in restriction of diastolic filling and cavity obliteration.

Valvar disease

Rheumatic heart disease may have declined in certain parts of the world, but it still represents an important cause of heart failure in India and other developing countries. In the Framingham study rheumatic heart disease accounted for heart failure in 2% of men and 3% of women, although the overall incidence of valvar disease has been steadily decreasing in the Framingham cohort over the past 30 years. Valve disease was thought to be the primary cause of heart failure in 10% of incident cases in the Bromley study, carried out in the late 1990s.

> It is important to diagnose valvular disease not only to establish aetiology but also because in some cases there are potentially other "curative" options (from the heart failure point of view)— for instance, surgery

Mitral regurgitation and aortic stenosis are the most common causes of heart failure secondary to valvar disease in developed countries. Mitral (and aortic) regurgitation leads to volume overload (increased preload), in contrast with aortic stenosis, which leads to pressure overload (increased afterload). The progression of heart failure in patients with valvar disease depends on the nature and extent of the valvar disease.

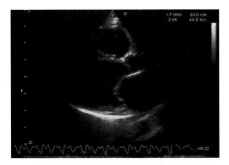
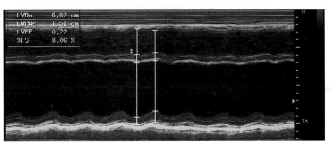

Two dimensional (long axis parasternal view) echocardiogram (top) and M mode echocardiogram (bottom) showing severely impaired left ventricular function in dilated cardiomyopathy

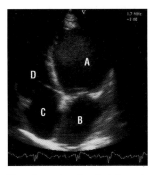

Two dimensional, apical, four chamber echocardiogram showing dilated cardiomyopathy. A = left ventricle; B = left atrium; C = right atrium; D = right ventricle

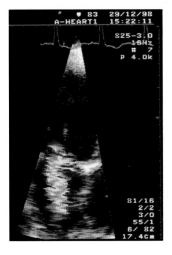

Color Doppler echocardiogram showing mitral regurgitation

ABC of heart failure

In aortic stenosis, heart failure develops at a relatively late stage and, without valve replacement, it is associated with a poor prognosis. In contrast, patients with chronic mitral (or aortic) regurgitation generally decline in a slower and more progressive manner.

Arrhythmias

Cardiac arrhythmias are more common in patients with heart failure and associated structural heart disease, including patients with hypertension and left ventricular hypertrophy.

Ventricular arrhythmias are also commonly seen in heart failure, leading to a sudden deterioration in some patients; such arrhythmias are a major cause of sudden death in those with heart failure, which is why implantable defibrillators are increasingly being used in such patients (see chapter 7).

Atrial fibrillation and heart failure often coexist, and this has been confirmed in large scale trials and smaller hospital based studies. In the Hillingdon heart failure study 30% of patients presenting for the first time with heart failure had atrial fibrillation, usually in association with other cardiac abnormalities, and over 60% of patients admitted urgently with atrial fibrillation to a Glasgow hospital had echocardiographic evidence of impaired left ventricular function.

Atrial fibrillation is more common with increasing severity of heart failure. Some studies have found that atrial fibrillation in patients with heart failure is associated with increased mortality, though the vasodilator heart failure trial (V-HeFT) failed to show an increase in major morbidity or mortality for patients with atrial fibrillation. In the stroke prevention in atrial fibrillation (SPAF) study, the presence of concomitant heart failure or left ventricular dysfunction increased the risk of stroke and thromboembolism in patients with atrial fibrillation. As this high risk of stroke is reduced by two thirds by anticoagulation with warfarin, it is essential that such high risk patients are identified and treated.

Alcohol and drugs

Alcohol has a direct toxic effect on the heart, which may lead to acute heart failure or heart failure as a result of arrhythmias, commonly atrial fibrillation. Alcohol can also lead to hypertension. Excessive chronic alcohol consumption also leads to dilated cardiomyopathy (alcoholic heart muscle disease). Alcohol is the identifiable cause of chronic heart failure in 2–3% of cases. Rarely, alcohol misuse may be associated with general nutritional deficiency and thiamine deficiency (beriberi).

Chemotherapeutic agents (such as doxorubicin) and antiviral drugs (such as zidovudine) have been implicated in heart failure through direct toxic effects on the myocardium.

Other causes

Infections may precipitate heart failure as a result of the toxic metabolic effects (relative hypoxia, acid base disturbance) in combination with peripheral vasodilation and tachycardia, leading to increased myocardial oxygen demand. Patients with chronic heart failure, like patients with most chronic illnesses, are particularly susceptible to viral and bacterial respiratory infections. Rarely, some viral infections (such as, coxsackie virus and echovirus) can cause a viral myocarditis.

"High output" heart failure is sometimes described in patients with severe anaemia and thyrotoxicosis, though it is

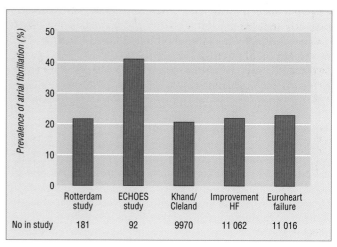

Prevalence of chronic atrial fibrillation in epidemiological studies and surveys. Adapted from Cleland JG, et al. *Heart Fail Rev* 2002;7:229–42

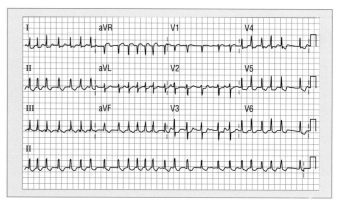

Electrocardiogram showing atrial fibrillation with a rapid ventricular response

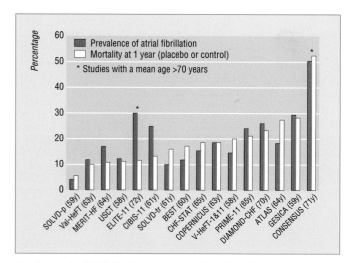

Prevalence of atrial fibrillation in pharmacological studies of chronic heart failure ranked according to one year mortality in placebo group as marker of severity of heart failure. Adapted from Cleland JG, et al. *Heart Fail Rev* 2002;7:229–42

debatable whether such a label should be used as the primary problem is not one of a failing heart. Myxoedema may present with heart failure as a result of myocardial involvement or secondary to a pericardial effusion.

A cardiomyopathy can be associated with pregnancy and the postpartum period, when it is referred to as "puerperal cardiomyopathy."

This chapter was adapted from the corresponding one in the first edition written by GYH Lip, CR Gibbs, and DG Beevers. Our colleagues' previous contribution is gratefully acknowledged.

Further reading

- Cowie MR, Wood DA, Coats AJS, Thompson SG, Poole-Wilson PA, Suresh V, et al. Incidence and aetiology of heart failure: a population-based study. *Eur Heart J* 1999;20:421–8.
- Fox KF, Cowie MR, Wood DA, Coats AJ, Gibbs JS, Underwood SR, et al. Coronary artery disease as the cause of incident heart failure in the population. *Eur Heart J* 2001;22:228–36.
- Levy D, Larson MG, Vasan RS, Kannel WB, Ho KKL. The progression from hypertension to congestive heart failure. *JAMA* 1996;275:1557–62.
- Oakley C. Aetiology, diagnosis, investigation, and management of cardiomyopathies. *BMJ* 1997;315:1520–4.
- Teerlink JR, Goldhaber SZ, Pfeffer MA. An overview of contemporary etiologies of congestive heart failure. *Am Heart J* 1991;121:1852–3.

3 Pathophysiology

Developments in our understanding of the pathophysiology of heart failure have been essential for recent therapeutic advances in this specialty

Heart failure is a multisystem disorder that is characterised by abnormalities of cardiac and skeletal muscle and renal function; stimulation of the sympathetic nervous system; and a complex pattern of neurohormonal changes.

Broadly, damage to the myocytes and extracellular matrix—after myocardial infarction or myocarditis, etc—results in changes in the size, shape, and function of the left ventricle and heart, commonly referred to as "myocardial remodelling". The latter results in electrical instability—precipitating arrhythmias, etc—as well as activating systemic processes causing sequelae in many other organs and tissues, as well as further damage to the heart. These vicious cycles lead to progressive worsening of the heart failure syndrome over time.

Myocardial systolic dysfunction

The primary abnormality in non-valvar heart failure is an impairment in left ventricular function, leading to a fall in cardiac output (in valvar disease, cardiac output also falls, even though ventricular function is preserved). The fall in cardiac output leads to activation of several neurohormonal compensatory mechanisms aimed at improving the mechanical environment of the heart. Activation of the sympathetic system, for example, tries to maintain cardiac output with an increase in heart rate, increased myocardial contractility, and peripheral vasoconstriction (increased catecholamines). Activation of the renin-angiotensin-aldosterone system (RAAS) also results in vasoconstriction (angiotensin) and an increase in blood volume, with retention of salt and water (aldosterone). Indeed, they each stimulate the actions of each, allowing for deleterious persistent or chronic overactivity of both. Concentrations of vasopressin and natriuretic peptides increase. There may also be progressive cardiac dilatation or alterations in cardiac structure (remodelling), or both.

After myocardial infarction

- Plasma concentration of norepinephrine (norepinephrine) is of prognostic value in patients early after myocardial infarction, predicting subsequent changes in left ventricular volume
- Natriuretic peptides have also been shown to predict outcome after myocardial infarction, though it is not clear whether the predictive value is additive to measurements of ventricular function

Neurohormonal activation

Chronic heart failure is associated with neurohormonal activation and alterations in autonomic control. Though these compensatory neurohormonal mechanisms provide valuable support for the heart in normal physiological circumstances, they also have a fundamental role in the development and subsequent progression of chronic heart failure.

Renin-angiotensin-aldosterone system
Stimulation of the RAAS leads to increased concentrations of renin, plasma angiotensin II, and aldosterone. Angiotensin II is

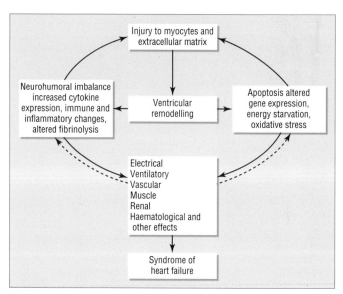

Pathophysiology of heart failure due to left ventricular systolic function. Adapted from McMurray J, et al. *Lancet* 2005;365:1877

Other hormonal mechanisms in chronic heart failure

- The arachidonic acid cascade leads to increased concentrations of prostaglandins (prostaglandin E_2 and prostaglandin I_2), which protect the glomerular microcirculation during renal vasoconstriction and maintain glomerular filtration by dilating afferent glomerular arterioles
- The kallikrein kinin system forms bradykinin, resulting in both natriuresis and vasodilatation, and stimulates the production of prostaglandins
- Circulating concentrations of the cytokine tumour necrosis factor α (TNF-α) are increased in cachectic patients with chronic heart failure. TNF-α has also been implicated in the development of endothelial abnormalities in patients with chronic heart failure

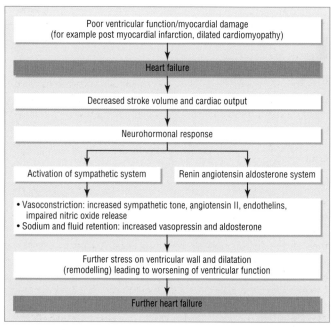

Neurohormonal mechanisms and compensatory mechanisms in heart failure

a potent vasoconstrictor of the renal (efferent arterioles) and systemic circulation, where it stimulates release of norepinephrine (norepinephrine) from sympathetic nerve terminals, inhibits vagal tone, and promotes the release of aldosterone. This leads to the retention of sodium and water and the increased excretion of potassium. In addition, angiotensin II has important effects on cardiac myocytes and may contribute to the endothelial dysfunction that is observed in chronic heart failure, and aldosterone can cause myocardial fibrosis and thereby impaired diastolic function.

Sympathetic nervous system

The sympathetic nervous system is activated in heart failure, via low and high pressure baroreceptors, as an early compensatory mechanism that provides inotropic support and maintains cardiac output. Chronic sympathetic activation, however, has deleterious effects, causing a further deterioration in cardiac function.

The earliest increase in sympathetic activity is detected in the heart, and this seems to precede the increase in sympathetic outflow to skeletal muscle and the kidneys that is present in advanced heart failure. Sustained sympathetic stimulation activates the RAAS and other neurohormones, leading to increased venous and arterial tone (and greater preload and afterload, respectively), increased plasma norepinephrine concentrations, progressive retention of salt and water, and oedema. Excessive sympathetic activity is also associated with cardiac myocyte apoptosis, hypertrophy, and focal myocardial necrosis.

In the long term, the ability of the myocardium to respond to chronic high concentrations of catecholamines is attenuated by a down regulation in β receptors, though this may be associated with baroreceptor dysfunction and a further increase in sympathetic activity. Indeed, abnormalities of baroreceptor function are well documented in chronic heart failure, along with reduced parasympathetic tone, leading to abnormal autonomic modulation of the sinus node. Moreover, a reduction in heart rate variability has consistently been observed in chronic heart failure as a result of predominantly sympathetic and reduced vagal modulation of the sinus node, which may be a prognostic marker in patients with chronic heart failure.

Natriuretic peptides

Several natriuretic peptides, of similar structure, have now been isolated and these exert a wide range of effects on the heart, kidneys, and central nervous system.

Atrial natriuretic peptide (ANP) is released from the atria in response to stretch, leading to natriuresis and vasodilatation. In humans, brain or b-type natriuretic peptide (BNP) is also released from the heart, predominantly from the ventricles, and its actions are similar to those of atrial natriuretic peptide. C-type natriuretic peptide and urodilatin are mainly secreted elsewhere.

ANP and BNP concentrations increase in response to volume expansion and pressure overload of the heart and act as physiological antagonists to the effects of angiotensin II on vascular tone, aldosterone secretion, and renal tubule sodium reabsorption. As the natriuretic peptides are important mediators, with increased circulating concentrations in patients with heart failure, interest has developed in both the diagnostic and prognostic potential of these peptides (see chapter 5). Intravenous nesiritide, synthetic recombinant BNP, has been shown to have benefits over traditional therapies in acutely decompensated heart failure, and is now commonly used in the US, although recently there have been worrying reports of increased mortality. Agents that inhibit the enzyme that

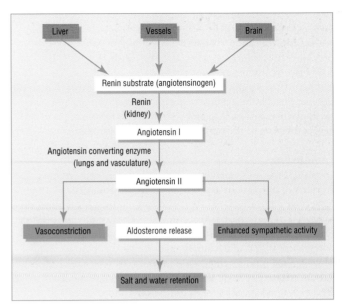

Renin-angiotensin-aldosterone axis in heart failure

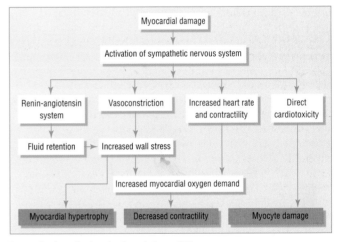

Sympathetic activation in chronic heart failure

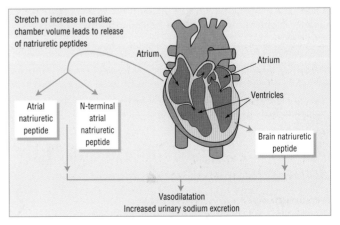

Effects of natriuretic peptides

metabolises atrial natriuretic peptide (neutral endopeptidase), such as omapatrilat, have also been developed, but this drug was withdrawn because of an excess of angio-oedema.

Antidiuretic hormone (vasopressin)

Antidiuretic hormone concentrations are also increased in severe chronic heart failure. High concentrations of the hormone are particularly common in patients on diuretic treatment, and this may contribute to the development of hyponatraemia.

Endothelins

Endothelin is secreted by vascular endothelial cells and is a potent vasoconstrictor peptide that has pronounced vasoconstrictor effects on the renal vasculature, promoting the retention of sodium. Importantly, the plasma concentration of endothelin-1 is of prognostic importance and is increased in proportion to the symptomatic and haemodynamic severity of heart failure. Endothelin concentration is also correlated with indices of severity such as the pulmonary artery capillary wedge pressure, need for admission to hospital, and death.

Because of the vasoconstrictor properties of endothelin, interest has developed in endothelin receptor antagonists as cardioprotective agents that inhibit endothelin mediated vascular and myocardial remodelling. As yet, however, trials of drugs such as bosentan have been disappointing, though in some patients with right heart failure secondary to primary pulmonary hypertension bosentan may be useful.

Patterns of neurohormonal activation and prognosis

Asymptomatic left ventricular dysfunction

Plasma norepinephrine (norepinephrine) concentrations increase early in the development of left ventricular dysfunction, and plasma renin activity usually increases in patients receiving diuretic treatment. Norepinephrine concentration in asymptomatic left ventricular dysfunction is a strong and independent predictor of the development of symptomatic chronic heart failure and long term mortality. Plasma concentrations of BNP and N-terminal pro-brain natriuretic peptide (NT-proBNP) also seem to be good indicators of asymptomatic left ventricular dysfunction and may be useful as an objective blood test in these patients.

Congestive heart failure

In severe untreated chronic heart failure, concentrations of renin, angiotensin II, aldosterone, norepinephrine, ANP, and BNP are all increased. Plasma concentrations of various neuroendocrine markers correlate with both the severity of heart failure and the long term prognosis. For example, raised plasma concentrations of BNP and NT-proBNP are independent predictors of mortality in patients with chronic heart failure. Patients with congestive heart failure and raised plasma norepinephrine concentrations also have a worse prognosis. In patients referred for assessment for heart transplantation, NT-proBNP concentration was a more powerful prognostic marker than the traditional measures of ejection fraction, peak oxygen uptake (VO_2 Max), or the composite heart failure survival score.

Other non-cardiac abnormalities in chronic heart failure

Vasculature

The vascular endothelium has an important role in the regulation of vascular tone, releasing relaxing and contracting

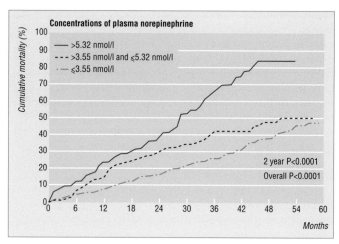

Norepinephrine concentrations and prognosis in chronic heart failure. Adapted from Cohn JN, et al. *N Engl J Med* 1984;311:819–23

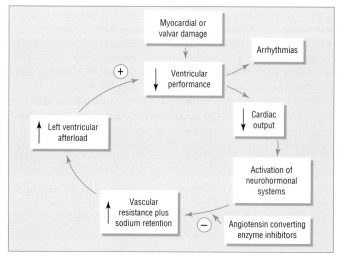

Effect of angiotensin converting inhibitors in heart failure

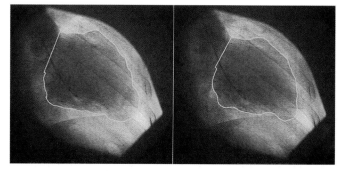

Contrast left ventriculogram in patient with poor systolic function (diastolic (left) and systolic (right) views)

factors under basal conditions or during exercise. The increased peripheral resistance in patients with chronic heart failure is related to the alterations in autonomic control, including heightened sympathetic tone, activation of the RAAS, increased endothelin concentrations, and impaired release of endothelium derived relaxing factor (or nitric oxide). There is emerging evidence that impaired endothelial function in chronic heart failure may be improved with exercise training and drug treatment, such as angiotensin converting enzyme inhibitors.

Changes in skeletal muscle

Considerable peripheral changes occur in the skeletal muscle of patients with chronic heart failure. These include a reduction in muscle mass and abnormalities in muscle structure, metabolism, and function. There is also reduced blood flow to active skeletal muscle, which is related to vasoconstriction and the loss in muscle mass. All these abnormalities in skeletal muscles, including respiratory muscles, contribute to the symptoms of fatigue, lethargy, and exercise intolerance that occur in chronic heart failure. Exercise rehabilitation has been shown to reverse many of these skeletal muscle changes.

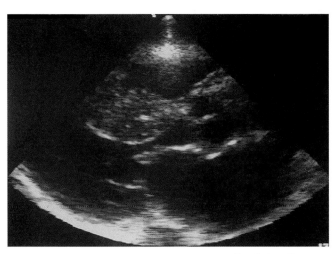

Two dimensional echocardiogram in a patient with hypertrophic cardiomyopathy showing asymmetrical septal hypertrophy

Diastolic dysfunction

Diastolic dysfunction results from impaired myocardial relaxation, with increased stiffness in the ventricular wall and reduced left ventricular compliance, leading to impairment of diastolic ventricular filling. Infiltrations, such as amyloid heart disease, are the best examples, though coronary artery disease, hypertension (with left ventricular hypertrophy), and hypertrophic cardiomyopathy are more common causes. Failure of the left ventricle to fill completely leads to a reduced cardiac output, and the increased filling pressure required can lead to pulmonary congestion, causing symptomatic heart failure.

The incidence and contribution of diastolic dysfunction remains controversial, though it has been estimated that 30–40% of patients with heart failure have normal ventricular systolic contraction. Indices of diastolic dysfunction can be obtained non-invasively with Doppler echocardiography or invasively with cardiac catheterisation and measurement of changes in left ventricular pressure. There is no agreement as to the most accurate index of left ventricular diastolic dysfunction, but the Doppler mitral inflow velocity profile is probably the most widely used.

Though pure forms exist, in most patients with heart failure both systolic and diastolic dysfunction can be present. Knowing about diastolic dysfunction, however, has little effect on management of most patients with chronic heart failure as there are still many uncertainties over its measurement and optimal management strategies.

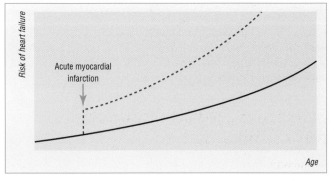

Contrast left ventriculogram in patient with hypertrophic cardiomyopathy (diastolic (left) and systolic (right) views)

Myocardial remodelling, hibernation, and stunning

Cardiac contractility is often impaired after extensive myocardial infarction, and neurohormonal activation leads to regional eccentric and concentric hypertrophy of the non-infarcted segment, with expansion (regional thinning and dilatation) of the infarct zone. This is known as remodelling. Particular risk factors for this development of progressive ventricular dilatation after a myocardial infarction include a large infarct, anterior infarctions, occlusion (or non-reperfusion) of the artery related to the infarct, and hypertension.

Risk of heart failure and relation with age and history of myocardial infarction

Myocardial dysfunction may also occur in response to "stunning" (postischaemic dysfunction), which describes delayed recovery of myocardial function despite restoration of coronary blood flow in the absence of irreversible damage. This is in contrast with "hibernating" myocardium, which describes persistent myocardial dysfunction at rest secondary to reduced myocardial perfusion, though cardiac myocytes remain viable and myocardial contraction may improve with revascularisation.

When stunning or hibernation occurs, viable myocardium retains responsiveness to inotropic stimulation, which can then be identified by resting and stress echocardiography, thallium scintigraphy, positron emission tomography, or magnetic resonance imaging with gadolinium. Revascularisation may improve the overall left ventricular function with potential beneficial effects on symptoms and prognosis.

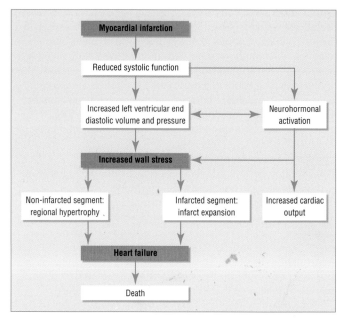

Process of ventricular remodelling. Adapted from McKay RG, et al. *Circulation* 1986;74:693–702

Further reading

- Bhatia G, Sosin M, Leahy JF, Connolly DL, Davis RC, Lip GY. Hibernating myocardium in heart failure. *Expert Rev Cardiovasc Ther* 2005;3:111–22.
- Gardner RS, Ozalp F, Murday AJ, Robb SD, McDonagh TA. N-terminal pro-brain natriuretic peptide. A new gold standard in predicting mortality in patients with advanced heart failure. *Eur Heart J* 2003;24:1735–43.
- McDonagh TA, Robb SD, Murdoch DR, Morton JJ, Ford I, Morrison CE, et al. Biochemical detection of left ventricular systolic dysfunction. *Lancet* 1998;351:9–13.
- Packer M. The neurohormonal hypothesis: a theory to explain the mechanisms of disease progression in heart failure. *J Am Coll Cardiol* 1992;20:248–54.
- Yusuf S, Pfeffer MA, Swedberg K, Granger CB, Held P, McMurray JJV, et al, for the CHARM investigators and committees. Effects of candesartan in patients with chronic heart failure and preserved left ventricular ejection fraction: the CHARM-preserved trial. *Lancet* 2003;362:777–81.

This chapter was adapted from the corresponding one in the first edition written by G Jackson, CR Gibbs, MK Davies, and GYH Lip. Our colleagues' previous contribution is gratefully acknowledged.

4 Clinical features and complications

Clinical features

Patients with heart failure present with various symptoms, most of which are non-specific. The common symptoms of congestive heart failure include fatigue, dyspnoea, swollen ankles, and exercise intolerance, or symptoms that relate to the underlying cause. The accuracy of diagnosis by presenting clinical features alone, however, is often inadequate, particularly in women and elderly or obese patients.

Symptoms
Dyspnoea
Breathlessness on exertion is a common presenting symptom in heart failure, though it is also a common (non-cardiac) symptom in the general population, particularly in patients with pulmonary disease. Dyspnoea is therefore moderately sensitive, but poorly specific, for the presence of heart failure. Orthopnoea is a more specific symptom, though it has a low sensitivity. Paroxysmal nocturnal dyspnoea results from increased left ventricular filling pressures (due to nocturnal fluid redistribution and enhanced renal reabsorption). Nocturnal ischaemic chest pain may also be a manifestation of heart failure so left ventricular systolic dysfunction should be excluded in patients with recurrent nocturnal angina.

Fatigue and lethargy
Fatigue and lethargy in chronic heart failure are, in part, related to abnormalities in skeletal muscle, with premature muscle lactate release, impaired muscle blood flow, deficient endothelial function, and abnormalities in skeletal muscle structure and function. Reduced cerebral blood flow, when accompanied by abnormal sleep patterns, may occasionally lead to somnolence and confusion in severe chronic heart failure. Disordered breathing patterns during sleep are increasingly recognised as being very common in patients with heart failure and can contribute to daytime symptoms of fatigue.

Oedema
Swelling of ankles and feet is another common presenting feature, though there are numerous non-cardiac causes of this symptom. Right heart failure may manifest as oedema, right hypochondrial pain (liver distension), abdominal swelling (ascites), loss of appetite, and, rarely, malabsorption (bowel oedema). An increase in weight may be associated with fluid retention, though cardiac cachexia and weight loss are important markers of advanced disease in some patients.

Physical signs
Physical examination has serious limitations as many patients, particularly those with less severe heart failure, have few abnormal signs. In addition, some physical signs are difficult to interpret and, if present, may occasionally be related to causes other than heart failure.

Oedema and tachycardia, for example, are too insensitive to have useful predictive value in the detection of early disease in the community, and though pulmonary crepitations may have a high diagnostic specificity they have a low sensitivity and predictive value. Indeed, the commonest cause of lower limb oedema in elderly people is immobility, and pulmonary

---

Symptoms and signs in heart failure

Symptoms	Signs
• Dyspnoea	• Tachycardia
• Orthopnoea	• Pulsus alternans
• Paroxysmal nocturnal dyspnoea	• Raised jugular venous pressure
	• Displaced apex beat
• Reduced exercise tolerance, lethargy fatigue	• Right ventricular heave
	• Crepitations or wheeze
• Nocturnal cough	• Third heart sound
• Wheeze	• Oedema
• Ankle swelling	• Hepatomegaly (tender)
• Anorexia	• Ascites
	• Cachexia and muscle wasting

Precipitating causes of heart failure
- Arrhythmias, especially atrial fibrillation
- Infections (especially pneumonia)
- Acute myocardial infarction
- Recurrent myocardial ischaemia
- Anaemia
- Alcohol excess
- Iatrogenic cause—for example, postoperative fluid replacement or administration of steroids or non-steroidal anti-inflammatory drugs
- Poor drug compliance, especially in antihypertensive treatment
- Thyroid disorders—for example, thyrotoxicosis
- Pulmonary embolism
- Pregnancy

Common causes of lower limb oedema
- Gravitational disorder—for example, immobility
- Congestive heart failure
- Venous insufficiency, thrombosis or obstruction, varicose veins
- Hypoproteinaemia—for example, nephrotic syndrome, liver disease
- Lymphatic obstruction
- Drugs—particularly calcium antagonists

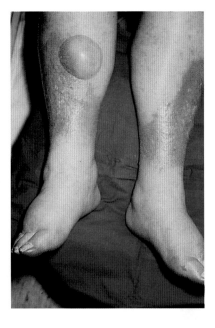

Gross oedema of the ankles, including bullae with serious exudates

ABC of heart failure

crepitations may reflect poor ventilation with infection, or pulmonary fibrosis, rather than heart failure. Jugular venous distension has a high specificity in diagnosing heart failure in patients who are known to have cardiac disease, though some patients, even with documented heart failure, do not have a raised venous pressure, especially if they are already on medication. The presence of a displaced apex beat in a patient with a history of myocardial infarction has a high positive predictive value. A third heart sound has a relatively high specificity, though its universal value is limited by a high interobserver variability, with interobserver agreement of less than 50% in non-specialists.

In patients with pre-existing chronic heart failure, other clinical features may be evident that point towards precipitating causes of acute heart failure or deteriorating heart failure. Common factors that may be obvious on clinical assessment and are associated with relapses in congestive heart failure include infections, arrhythmias, continued or recurrent myocardial ischaemia, and anaemia.

Signs and symptoms are only a part of the diagnostic investigation of a patient with heart failure, which should be complemented by additional investigations, as discussed in chapter 5. The European Society of Cardiology has recommended an algorithm for the diagnosis of heart failure.

Clinical diagnosis and clinical scoring systems

Several epidemiological studies, including the Framingham heart study, have used clinical scoring systems to define heart failure, though the use of these systems is not recommended for routine clinical practice.

In a patient with appropriate symptoms and several physical signs, including a displaced apex beat, raised venous pressure, oedema, and a third heart sound, the clinical diagnosis of heart failure may be made with some confidence. However, the clinical suspicion of heart failure should also be confirmed with objective investigations and the demonstration of cardiac dysfunction at rest. It is important to note that in some patients, exercise-induced myocardial ischaemia may lead to a rise in ventricular filling pressures and a fall in cardiac output, leading to symptoms of heart failure during exertion. It should be noted that a clinical response to treatment directed at heart failure alone is not sufficient for diagnosis, but the patient should show improvement in symptoms and/or signs in response to those therapies in which a relatively fast symptomatic improvement could be anticipated (for example, diuretic or nitrates).

Right and left heart failure refer to syndromes presenting predominantly with congestion of the systemic or pulmonary veins. High and low output, forward and backward, overt, treated, and congestive are other descriptive terms still in occasional use; but these are of little use in determining modern treatment for heart failure.

Mild, moderate, or severe heart failure is used as a clinical symptomatic description. Asymptomatic left ventricular systolic dysfunction is considered a precursor of symptomatic chronic heart failure and is associated with high mortality.

Classification

Symptoms and exercise capacity are used to classify the severity of heart failure and monitor the response to treatment. The classification of the New York Heart Association (NYHA) is used widely, though outcome in heart failure is best determined not only by symptoms (NYHA class) but also by echocardiographic criteria. As the disease is progressive, the

European Society of Cardiology guidelines for diagnosis of heart failure

Essential features
- Symptoms of heart failure (for example, breathlessness, fatigue)
- Objective evidence of cardiac dysfunction (at rest)

Non-essential features
- Response to treatment directed towards heart failure (in cases where the diagnosis is in doubt)

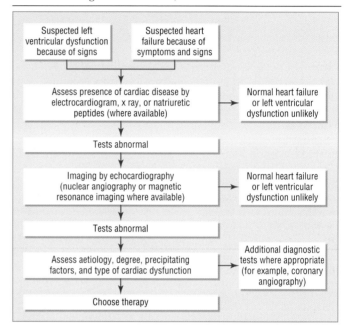

Algorithm diagnosis of heart failure, as recommended by the European Society of Cardiology

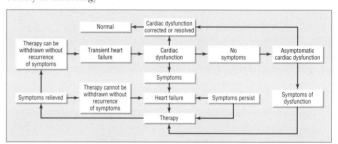

Distinctions between cardiac dysfunction, persistent heart failure, heart failure that has been rendered asymptomatic by therapy, and transient heart failure Adapted from Task force for the diagnosis and treatment of chronic heart failure. *Eur Heart J* 2005;26:1115–40

NYHA classification of heart failure

Class I: asymptomatic
No limitation of normal physical activity despite presence of heart disease. This can be suspected only if there is a history of heart disease that is confirmed by investigations—for example, echocardiography

Class II: "mild"
Slight limitation of physical activity. At the milder end of class II, more strenuous activity causes shortness of breath—for example, walking on steep inclines and several flights of steps. Patients in this group can continue to have an almost normal lifestyle and employment. At the more severe end, patients can be short of breath on one flight of stairs and be unable to work except at a desk, calling into question the label "mild"

Class III: moderate
Marked limitation of activity with symptoms even on mild physical exertion. Walking on the flat indoors and washing and dressing produce symptoms

Class IV: severe
Unable to carry out any physical activity without symptoms. Patients are breathless at rest and mostly housebound

importance of early treatment, in an attempt to prevent progression to more severe disease, cannot be overemphasised.

Complications

Arrhythmias
Atrial fibrillation
Atrial fibrillation is present in about a third (range 10–50%) of patients with chronic heart failure and may represent either a cause or a consequence of heart failure. The onset of atrial fibrillation with a rapid ventricular response may precipitate overt heart failure, particularly in patients with pre-existing ventricular dysfunction and mitral valve disease. Sometimes, the onset of atrial fibrillation itself—irrespective of rate—may precipitate heart failure, especially in the presence of diastolic dysfunction, secondary to hypertensive left ventricular hypertrophy.

Predisposing causes for atrial fibrillation should be considered, including lung disease, thyrotoxicosis, and sinus node disease. Importantly, sinus node disease may be associated with bradycardias, which might be exacerbated by antiarrhythmic treatment.

Atrial fibrillation that occurs with severe left ventricular dysfunction after myocardial infarction is associated with a poor prognosis. In addition, patients with heart failure and atrial fibrillation are at particularly high risk of stroke and other thromboembolic complications. In these patients anticoagulation with warfarin can reduce risk by two thirds.

Ventricular arrhythmias
Malignant ventricular arrhythmias are common in end stage heart failure. For example, sustained monomorphic ventricular tachycardia occurs in up to 10% of patients with advanced heart failure who are referred for cardiac transplantation. In patients with ischaemic heart disease these arrhythmias often have re-entrant mechanisms in scarred myocardial tissue. An episode of sustained ventricular tachycardia indicates a high risk for recurrent ventricular arrhythmias and sudden cardiac death.

Sustained polymorphic ventricular tachycardia and torsades de pointes are more likely to occur in the presence of precipitating or aggravating factors, including electrolyte disturbance (for example, hypokalaemia or hyperkalaemia, hypomagnesaemia), prolonged QT interval, digoxin toxicity, drugs causing electrical instability (for example, antiarrhythmic drugs, antidepressants), and continued or recurrent myocardial ischaemia. β blockers are useful for treating arrhythmias, and these agents (for example, bisoprolol, metoprolol, carvedilol) are increasingly used as standard treatment in patients with heart failure. Implantable cardiac defibrillators have made a great impact on management (see chapter 7).

Stroke and thromboembolism
Congestive heart failure predisposes patients to stroke and thromboembolism, with an overall estimated annual incidence of about 2%. Factors contributing to the increased thromboembolic risk in patients with heart failure include low cardiac output (with relative stasis of blood in dilated cardiac chambers), regional abnormalities in wall motion (including formation of a left ventricular aneurysm), and associated atrial fibrillation. Though the prevalence of atrial fibrillation in some of the earlier observational studies was between 12% and 36%—which may have accounted for some of the thromboembolic events—patients with chronic heart failure who remain in sinus rhythm are also at an increased risk of stroke and venous thromboembolism. Patients with heart failure and chronic venous insufficiency may also be immobile, and this contributes to their increased risk of thrombosis, including deep venous thrombosis and pulmonary embolism.

Complications of heart failure
- *Arrhythmias*—atrial fibrillation; ventricular arrhythmias (ventricular tachycardia, ventricular fibrillation); bradyarrhythmias
- *Thromboembolism*—stroke; peripheral embolism; deep venous thrombosis; pulmonary embolism
- *Gastrointestinal*—hepatic congestion and hepatic dysfunction; malabsorption
- *Musculoskeletal*—muscle wasting
- *Respiratory*—pulmonary congestion; respiratory muscle weakness; pulmonary hypertension (rare)

Predisposing factors for ventricular arrhythmias
- Recurrent or continued coronary ischaemia
- Recurrent myocardial infarction
- Hypokalaemia and hyperkalaemia
- Hypomagnesaemia
- Psychotropic drugs—for example, tricyclic antidepressants
- Digoxin (leading to toxicity)
- Antiarrhythmic drugs that may be cardiodepressant (negative inotropism) and proarrhythmic

---

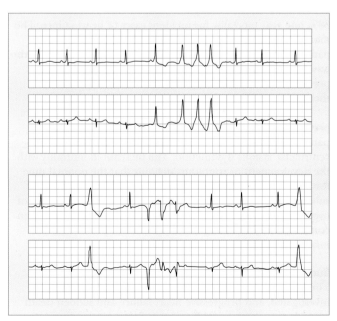

24 Hour Holter tracing showing frequent ventricular extrasystoles

5 Investigation

Clinical assessment is mandatory before detailed investigations are conducted in patients with suspected heart failure, though specific clinical features are often absent and the condition can be diagnosed accurately only in conjunction with more objective investigation, particularly echocardiography. Though echocardiography is increasingly widely available, investigations before referral include 12 lead electrocardiography, chest radiography, renal chemistry, and natriuretic peptide analysis (brain or b-type natriuretic peptide (BNP) or its precursor, N-terminal pro-brain natriuretic peptide (NT-proBNP)).

12 lead electrocardiography

The 12 lead electrocardiogram (ECG) tracing is abnormal in most patients with heart failure, especially those with more severe disease. Common abnormalities include bundle branch block, Q waves, abnormalities in the T wave and ST segment, left ventricular hypertrophy, and atrial fibrillation. A cardiac cause of dyspnoea is unlikely if the BNP level (in a patient not being treated) and an electrocardiographic tracing are normal.

In patients with symptoms (palpitations or dizziness), 24 hour ECG (Holter) monitoring or a cardiomemo device can detect paroxysmal arrhythmias such as ventricular extrasystoles, sustained or non-sustained ventricular tachycardia, and abnormal atrial rhythms (extrasystoles, supraventricular tachycardia, and paroxysmal atrial fibrillation). Asymptomatic arrhythmias are common in 24 hour monitoring in patients with heart failure.

Echocardiography

Echocardiography is the single most useful non-invasive test in the assessment of left ventricular function; ideally it should be conducted in all patients with suspected heart failure. Though clinical assessment, when combined with a chest x ray examination and electrocardiography, allows a preliminary diagnosis of heart failure, echocardiography provides an objective assessment of cardiac structure and function and defines the aetiology, which may not be otherwise apparent. Left ventricular dilatation and impairment of contraction is observed in patients with systolic dysfunction related to ischaemic heart disease (where an abnormality in regional wall motion may be detected) or in dilated cardiomyopathy (with global impairment of systolic contraction).

A quantitative measurement can be obtained from calculation of the left ventricular ejection fraction. This is the stroke volume (the difference between the end diastolic and end systolic volumes) expressed as a percentage of the left ventricular end diastolic volume. Measurements, and the assessment of left ventricular function, are less reliable in the presence of atrial fibrillation. The left ventricular ejection fraction has been correlated with outcome and survival in patients with heart failure, though the assessment may be more difficult in patients with abnormalities in regional wall motion. Regional abnormalities can also be quantified into a wall motion index, though in practice the assessment of systolic function is often based on visual assessment and the observer's experience of normal and abnormal contractile function. These

---

Investigations if heart failure is suspected

Initial investigations
- Electrocardiography
- Natriuretic peptide (where available; less useful if patient on treatment already)
- Echocardiography, including Doppler studies
- Full blood count
- Serum biochemistry, including renal function and glucose concentrations, liver function tests, lipids, and thyroid function tests
- Cardiac enzymes (only if recent infarction is suspected)

Other investigations
- Chest x ray
- Radionuclide imaging
- Cardiopulmonary exercise testing
- Cardiac catheterisation
- Myocardial biopsy—for example, in suspected myocarditis

Value of electrocardiography* in identifying heart failure resulting from left ventricular systolic dysfunction

Sensitivity	94%
Specificity	61%
Positive predictive value	35%
Negative predictive value	98%

*Electrocardiographic abnormalities are defined as atrial fibrillation, evidence of previous myocardial infarction, left ventricular hypertrophy, bundle branch block, and left axis deviation.
Adapted from Davie AP, et al. *BMJ* 1996;312:222

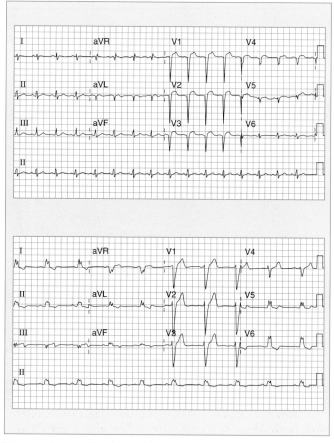

Electrocardiograms showing previous anterior myocardial infarction with Q waves in anteroseptal leads (top) and left bundle branch block (bottom)

abnormalities are described as hypokinetic (reduced systolic contraction), akinetic (no systolic contraction), dyskinetic (abnormal movement in systole), and aneurysmal (abnormal movement in systole and diastole), and refer to 16 defined segments of the left ventricle. Echocardiography may also show other abnormalities, including valvar disease, left ventricular aneurysm, intracardiac thrombus, and pericardial disease.

Mitral incompetence is commonly identified on echocardiography in patients with heart failure as a result of ventricular and annular dilatation ("functional" mitral incompetence), and this must be distinguished from mitral incompetence related to primary valve disease. Two dimensional echocardiography allows the assessment of valve structure and identifies thickening of cusps, leaflet prolapse, cusp fusion, and calcification. Doppler echocardiography allows the quantitative assessment of flow across valves and the identification of valve stenosis, in addition to the assessment of right ventricular systolic pressures and allowing the indirect diagnosis of pulmonary hypertension. Doppler studies have been used in the assessment of diastolic function, though there is no single reliable echocardiographic measure of diastolic dysfunction. Colour flow Doppler techniques are particularly sensitive in detecting the direction of blood flow and the presence of valve incompetence.

Advances in echocardiography include the use of contrast agents for visualisation of the walls of the left ventricle in more detail (in about 10% of patients satisfactory images cannot be obtained with standard transthoracic echocardiography). Transoesophageal echocardiography allows the detailed assessment of the atria, valves, pulmonary veins, and any ardiac masses, including thrombi. Tissue Doppler indices may also provide more useful measures of diastolic function.

The logistic and economic aspects of large scale screening with echocardiography have been debated, but the development of open access echocardiography heart failure services for general practitioners and the availability of proved treatments for heart failure that improve prognosis, such as angiotensin converting enzyme inhibitors, highlight the importance of an agreed strategy for such assessment of these patients.

Haematology and biochemistry

Routine haematology and biochemistry investigations are recommended to exclude anaemia as a cause of breathlessness and high output heart failure and to exclude important pre-existing metabolic abnormalities. Anaemia is also common in moderate to severe heart failure, and recent studies suggest a prognostic implication of such a finding.

Cardiac iron overload is a rare but treatable cause of systolic dysfunction, and therefore a haemochromatosis screen (serum iron, transferring, and ferritin) should be performed if aetiology is not obvious, for example, large Q wave infarction.

In mild and moderate heart failure, renal function and electrolytes are usually normal. In severe heart failure, however, as a result of reduced renal perfusion, high dose diuretics, sodium restriction, and activation of the neurohormonal mechanisms (including vasopressin), there is an inability to excrete water, and dilutional hyponatraemia may be present.

Hyponatraemia is a marker of the severity of chronic heart failure

A baseline assessment of renal function is important before treatment is started as the renal blood flow and the glomerular filtration rate fall in severe congestive heart failure. Baseline serum creatinine concentrations are important: increasing

A normal ECG suggests that the diagnosis of chronic heart failure should be carefully reviewed

Stress studies use graded physical exercise or pharmacological stress with agents such as dobutamine. Stress echocardiography is emerging as a useful technique for assessing reversibility of myocardial ischaemia and also myocardial viability in patients with coronary artery disease

The role echocardiography in guiding to management
- Identification of impaired systolic function for decision on treatment with angiotensin converting enzyme inhibitors
- Identification of diastolic dysfunction or predominantly right ventricular dysfunction
- Identification and assessment of valvar disease
- Assessment of embolic risk (severe left ventricular impairment with mural thrombus)

Who should undergo echocardiography
- Almost all patients with symptoms or signs of heart failure
- Symptoms of breathlessness in association with signs of a murmur
- Dyspnoea associated with atrial fibrillation
- Patients at "high risk" for left ventricular dysfunction—for example, those with anterior myocardial infarction, poorly controlled hypertension, or arrhythmias

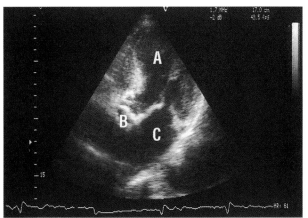

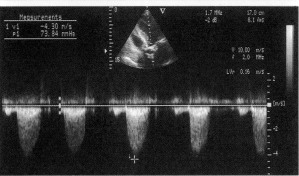

Transthoracic echocardiograms: two dimensional apical view (top) and Doppler studies (bottom) showing severe calcific stenosis, with an estimated aortic gradient of over 70 mm Hg (A = left ventricle, B = aortic valve, and C = left atrium)

creatinine concentrations may occur after the start of treatment, particularly in patients who are receiving angiotensin converting enzyme inhibitors and high doses of diuretics and in patients with renal artery stenosis. Proteinuria is a common finding in severe congestive heart failure.

Hypokalaemia occurs when high dose diuretics are used without potassium supplementation or potassium sparing agents. Hyperkalaemia can also occur in severe congestive heart failure with a low glomerular filtration rate, particularly with the concurrent use of angiotensin converting enzyme inhibitors and potassium sparing diuretics, including spironolactone. Both hypokalaemia and hyperkalaemia increase the risk of cardiac arrhythmias; hypomagnesaemia, which is associated with long term diuretic treatment, increases the risk of ventricular arrhythmias. Liver function tests (serum bilirubin, aspartate aminotransferase, and lactate dehydrogenase) are often abnormal in advanced congestive heart failure, as a result of hepatic congestion. Thyroid function tests are also recommended in all patients in view of the association between thyroid disease and the heart.

Chest x ray examination

The chest x ray examination has been regarded as a routine investigation for patients with suspected heart failure, but patients are increasingly being diagnosed and managed without it. Indeed, its greatest role may now be in the diagnosis of other causes of dyspnoea—for example, lung tumours or emphysema.

Cardiac enlargement (cardiothoracic ratio >50%) may be present, but there is a poor correlation between the cardiothoracic ratio and left ventricular function. The presence of cardiomegaly depends on both the severity of haemodynamic disturbance and its duration: cardiomegaly is often absent, for example, in acute left ventricular failure secondary to acute myocardial infarction, acute valvar regurgitation, or an acquired ventricular septal defect. An increased cardiothoracic ratio may be related to left or right ventricular dilatation, left ventricular hypertrophy, and occasionally a pericardial effusion, particularly if the cardiac silhouette has a globular appearance. Echocardiography is required to distinguish reliably between these different causes, which is why it has become the investigation of choice.

In left sided failure, pulmonary venous congestion occurs, initially in the upper zones (upper lobe diversion or congestion). When the pulmonary venous pressure increases further, usually above 20 mm Hg, fluid may be present in the horizontal fissure and septal (Kerly B) lines may be seen, with blunting of the costophrenic angles. In the presence of pulmonary venous pressures above 25 mm Hg, frank pulmonary oedema occurs, with a "bat's wing" appearance in the lungs. In addition, pleural effusions occur. Nevertheless, it is not possible to distinguish, when viewed in isolation, whether pulmonary congestion is related to cardiac or non-cardiac causes (such as renal disease, drugs). Rarely, chest radiography may also show valvar calcification, a left ventricular aneurysm, and the typical pericardial calcification of constrictive pericarditis.

Natriuretic peptides—BNP and NT-proBNP

At best only about a third of patients referred to diagnostic heart failure clinics and open access echocardiography services with suspected heart failure have the diagnosis confirmed after

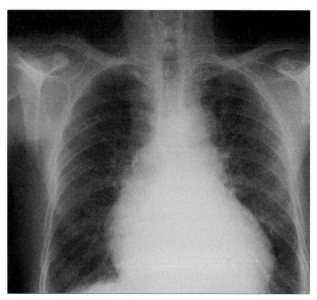

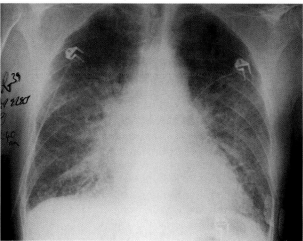

Chest radiographs showing gross cardiomegaly in patient with dilated cardiomyopathy (top); cardiomegaly and pulmonary congestion with fluid in horizontal fissure (bottom)

One of the key findings of studies in both the diagnostic clinic and emergency room settings is that low concentrations of BNP and NT-proBNP make the diagnosis of heart failure unlikely. By testing for BNP before referral it may be possible to avoid 25–30% of outpatient echocardiograms in this setting. Studies suggest that the sensitivity of BNP testing with a low cut-off level is about 97%; the "missed" cases will be those with a relatively good prognosis.

objective testing. In those presenting to emergency departments with acute shortness of breath, about half have heart failure. Because echocardiography is a scarce resource, there has been much interest in the use of biochemical markers to aid in the diagnosis of congestive heart failure. BNP, and its precursor molecule's metabolite, NT-proBNP, are produced in response to stretch of the cardiac ventricles and concentrations correlate with the severity of heart failure and prognosis.

In the emergency room setting, the "breathing not properly" study showed that rapid BNP testing was found to be highly predictive of heart failure and was more accurate than any clinical history or examination features or conventional laboratory analyses. Because of the severe acute stress on the cardiac ventricles in acute heart failure, BNP testing is particularly useful in this setting for distinguishing heart failure from other causes of acute dyspnoea.

The current evidence suggests that both BNP and NT-proBNP assays have similar sensitivity and specificity for heart failure and both tests have been used in the outpatient referral setting and the emergency room with similar results.

BNP and NT-proBNP are powerful predictors of mortality in several settings, and in patients referred to a cardiac transplantation centre, NT-proBNP was found to be a more powerful predictor of adverse outcome than traditional expensive and invasive tests such as VO_2 Max and right heart catheterisation. In determining who should be considered for heart transplantation, and also in other circumstances for terminal care, testing therefore has a potentially key role.

We cannot be sure how BNP performs diagnostically in large groups of patients with heart failure who are on treatment, and in such patients its diagnostic accuracy may fall and values be misleadingly low because of adequate and appropriate treatment. Furthermore we are uncertain how BNP measurement performs in heart failure associated with valvular disease where the ventricle is normal and underfilled (for example, mitral stenosis).

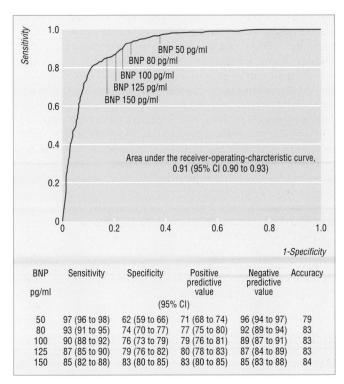

BNP pg/ml	Sensitivity	Specificity	Positive predictive value	Negative predictive value	Accuracy
		(95% CI)			
50	97 (96 to 98)	62 (59 to 66)	71 (68 to 74)	96 (94 to 97)	79
80	93 (91 to 95)	74 (70 to 77)	77 (75 to 80)	92 (89 to 94)	83
100	90 (88 to 92)	76 (73 to 79)	79 (76 to 81)	89 (87 to 91)	83
125	87 (85 to 90)	79 (76 to 82)	80 (78 to 83)	87 (84 to 89)	83
150	85 (82 to 88)	83 (80 to 85)	83 (80 to 85)	85 (83 to 88)	84

Various cut-off levels in B-type natriuretic peptide (BNP) in differentiating between dyspnoea due to congestive heart failure and dyspnoea due to other causes. Adapted from Maisel AS, et al. *N Engl J Med* 2002;161–7

> **Coronary angiography is still the ideal treatment for accurate anatomical assessment of the coronary arteries. Multislice computed tomography and magnetic resonance imaging hold promise for non-invasive assessment in the future**

Angiography, cardiac catheterisation, and myocardial biopsy

Angiography should be considered in patients with recurrent ischaemic chest pain associated with heart failure and those with evidence of severe reversible ischaemia or hibernating myocardium, or when the cause is in doubt. Coronary angiography is also the most reliable way of distinguishing between ischaemic heart failure and dilated cardiomyopathy, though magnetic resonance imaging with gadolinium enhancement is gaining in popularity. Myocardial biopsy can be valuable where there doubt about the diagnosis—for example, in restrictive and infiltrating cardiomyopathies (amyloid heart disease, sarcoidosis), myocarditis, and pericardial disease. Left ventricular angiography can show global or segmental impairment of function and assess end diastolic pressures, and right heart catheterisation allows an assessment of the right sided pressures (right atrium, right ventricle, and pulmonary arteries) and pulmonary artery capillary wedge pressure, in addition to oxygen saturations.

Radionuclide methods

Radionuclide imaging—or multigated ventriculography—allows the assessment of global left and right ventricular function. Images may be obtained in patients in whom echocardiography

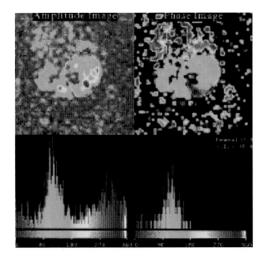

Multigated ventriculography scan in patient with history of extensive myocardial infarction and coronary bypass grafting (left ventricular ejection fraction of 30%)

is not possible. The most common method labels red cells with technetium-99 m and acquires 16 or 32 frames per heart beat by synchronising ("gating") imaging with electrocardiography. This allows the assessment of ejection fraction, systolic filling rate, diastolic emptying rate, and abnormalities in wall motion. These variables can be assessed, if necessary, during rest and exercise; this method is ideal for the serial reassessment of ejection fraction but does expose the patient to radiation.

Radionuclide studies are also valuable for assessing myocardial perfusion and the presence or extent of coronary ischaemia, including myocardial stunning and hibernating myocardium.

Magnetic resonance imaging

Magnetic resonance imaging is a useful for investigating left ventricular function and valvular disease in those who are poor echocardiographic subjects. It is non-invasive and does not involve ionising radiation. It is useful in studying dyssynchrony in possible candidates for cardiac resynchronisation therapy and in determining the aetiology of heart failure and if akinetic or severely hypokinetic areas of myocardium are viable but hibernating or irreversibly scarred.

Pulmonary function tests

Objective measurement of lung function can exclude respiratory causes of breathlessness, though respiratory and cardiac disease commonly coexist. Peak expiratory flow rate and forced expiratory volume in one second are reduced in heart failure, though lass so than in severe chronic obstructive pulmonary disease. In patients with severe breathlessness and wheeze, a peak expiratory flow rate of $<200\,1/min$ suggests reversible airways disease not acute left ventricular failure.

Since the routine use of β blockers, spirometry has become an increasingly important investigation in patients with known heart failure. Many patients are prescribed inhaled bronchodilators for their breathlessness, even though it is in fact caused by heart failure, and reversible airflow limitation needs to be excluded so that such patients can reap the benefits of β blockers. Patients with chronic lung disease and fixed airflow obstruction can be given β blockers, with caution.

Cardiopulmonary exercise testing

- Exercise tolerance is reduced in patients with heart failure, regardless of method of assessment
- Assessment methods include a treadmill test, cycle ergometry, a six minute walking test, or pedometry measurements
- Exercise testing is not routinely performed for all patients with congestive heart failure but it may be valuable in identifying substantial residual ischaemia, thus leading to more detailed investigation
- Respiratory physiological measurements may be made during exercise, and most cardiac transplant centres use data obtained at cardiopulmonary exercise testing to aid the selection of patients for transplantation
- The maximum oxygen consumption is the value at which consumption remains stable despite increasing exercise, and it represents the upper limit of aerobic exercise tolerance
- The maximum oxygen consumption and carbon dioxide production correlate well with the severity of heart failure
- The maximum oxygen consumption has also been independently related to long term prognosis, especially in patients with severe left ventricular dysfunction

Further reading

- Cheeseman MG, Leech G, Chambers J, Monaghan MJ, Nihoyannopoulos P. Central role of echocardiography in the diagnosis and assessment of heart failure. *Heart* 1998;80:Sl–5.
- Dargie HJ, McMurray JVV. Diagnosis and management of heart failure. *BMJ* 1994:308:321–8.
- Maisel AS, Krishnaswamy P, Nowk RM, McCord J, Hollander JE, Duc P, et al, for the Breathing Not Properly Multinational Study Investigators. Rapid measurement of B-type natriuretic peptide in the emergency diagnosis of heart failure. *N Engl J Med* 2002;347:161–7.
- Schiller NB, Foster E. Analysis of left ventricular systolic function. *Heart* 1996;75(suppl 2):17–26.
- Swedberg K, Cleland J, Dargie H, Drexler H, Follath F, et al. Guidelines for the diagnosis and treatment of chronic heart failure: executive summary (update 2005): the task force for the diagnosis and treatment of chronic heart failure of the European Society of Cardiology. *Eur Heart J* 2005;26:1115–40.

This chapter was adapted from the corresponding one in the first edition written by MK Davies, CR Gibbs, and GYH Lip. Our colleague's previous contribution is gratefully acknowledged.

Assessment for the investigation and diagnosis of heart failure (adapted with permission from the Task Force on Heart Failure of the European Society of Cardiology, *Eur Heart J* 1995;16:741–51)

Assessments	Diagnosis of heart failure			Suggests alternative or additional disease
	Necessary	Supports	Opposes	
Symptoms of heart failure	++		++ (if absent)	
Signs of heart failure		++	+ (if absent)	
Response to treatment		++	++ (if absent)	
Electrocardiography			++ (if normal)	
Chest radiography (cardiac dysfunction)		++	+ (if normal)	Pulmonary
Echocardiography (cardiac dysfunction)	++		++ (if absent)	
Haematology				Anaemia
Biochemistry (renal, liver function, and thyroid function tests)				Renal, liver, thyroid
Urine analysis				Renal
Pulmonary function tests				Pulmonary

++ = great importance; + = some importance.

6 Non-drug management

Approaches to the management of heart failure can be both non-pharmacological and pharmacological; each approach complements the other. Stages in the development of heart failure necessitate different approaches to management and recommendations for non-pharmacological and pharmacological treatment by stage.

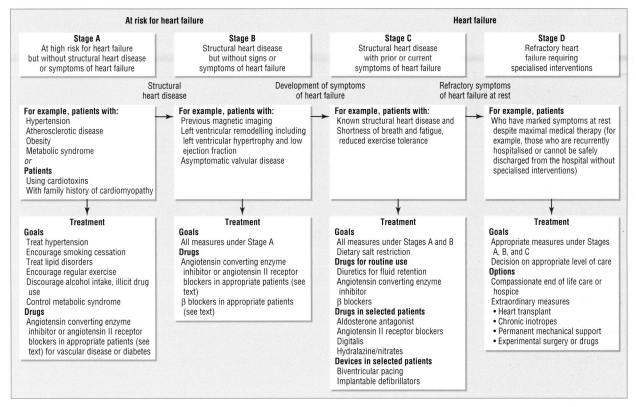

At risk for heart failure		Heart failure	
Stage A At high risk for heart failure but without structural heart disease or symptoms of heart failure	**Stage B** Structural heart disease but without signs or symptoms of heart failure	**Stage C** Structural heart disease with prior or current symptoms of heart failure	**Stage D** Refractory heart failure requiring specialised interventions
	Structural heart disease →	Development of symptoms of heart failure →	Refractory symptoms of heart failure at rest →
For example, patients with: Hypertension Atherosclerotic disease Obesity Metabolic syndrome *or* **Patients** Using cardiotoxins With family history of cardiomyopathy	**For example, patients with:** Previous magnetic imaging Left ventricular remodelling including left ventricular hypertrophy and low ejection fraction Asymptomatic valvular disease	**For example, patients with:** Known structural heart disease and Shortness of breath and fatigue, reduced exercise tolerance	**For example, patients** Who have marked symptoms at rest despite maximal medical therapy (for example, those who are recurrently hospitalised or cannot be safely discharged from the hospital without specialised interventions)
Treatment **Goals** Treat hypertension Encourage smoking cessation Treat lipid disorders Encourage regular exercise Discourage alcohol intake, illicit drug use Control metabolic syndrome **Drugs** Angiotensin converting enzyme inhibitor or angiotensin II receptor blockers in appropriate patients (see text) for vascular disease or diabetes	**Treatment** **Goals** All measures under Stage A **Drugs** Angiotensin converting enzyme inhibitor or angiotensin II receptor blockers in appropriate patients (see text) β blockers in appropriate patients (see text)	**Treatment** **Goals** All measures under Stages A and B Dietary salt restriction **Drugs for routine use** Diuretics for fluid retention Angiotensin converting enzyme inhibitor β blockers **Drugs in selected patients** Aldosterone antagonist Angiotensin II receptor blockers Digitalis Hydralazine/nitrates **Devices in selected patients** Biventricular pacing Implantable defibrillators	**Treatment** **Goals** Appropriate measures under Stages A, B, and C Decision on appropriate level of care **Options** Compassionate end of life care or hospice Extraordinary measures • Heart transplant • Chronic inotropes • Permanent mechanical support • Experimental surgery or drugs

Stages in the development of heart failure with recommended treatment by stage. Adapted from Hunt SA, et al. American College of Cardiology, www.acc.org/clinical/guidelines/failure/index.pdf

Counselling and education of patients

Effective counselling and education of patients, and of the relatives or carers, is important and may enhance long term adherence to management strategies. Simple explanations about the symptoms and signs of heart failure, including details of drug and other treatment strategies, are valuable. Emphasis should be placed on self help strategies for each patient; these should include information on the need to adhere to drug treatment. Some patients can be instructed on how to monitor their weight at home on a daily basis and how to adjust the dose of diuretics as advised; sudden weight increases (>2 kg in one to three days), for example, should alert a patient to alter his or her treatment or seek advice. As discussed in chapter 11, this might be best from a nurse specialist.

Lifestyle measures

Urging patients to alter their lifestyle is important in the management of chronic heart failure. Social activities should be encouraged, however, and care should be taken to ensure that patients avoid social isolation. If possible, they should continue

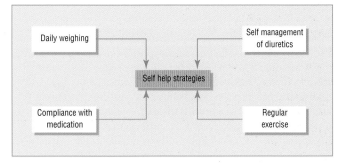

Self help strategies for patients with heart failure

their regular work, with adaptations to accommodate a reduced physical capacity when appropriate.

Salt and fluid restriction

No randomised studies have examined the role of salt restriction in congestive heart failure. Nevertheless restriction to about 2 g of sodium a day may be useful as an adjunct to treatment with high dose diuretics, particularly if the condition is advanced. In general, patients should be advised that they should avoid foods that are rich in salt and not to add salt to their food at the table.

Fluid restriction (1.5–2 litres daily) should be considered in patients with severe symptoms, those requiring high dose diuretics, and those with a tendency towards excessive fluid intake. High fluid intake negates the positive effects of diuretics and induces hyponatraemia.

Contraceptive advice

While heart failure due to ischaemic heart disease is rare in pre-menopausal women, dilated cardiomyopathy and myocarditis do occur and the condition of pregnancy-induced cardiomyopathy is rare but well recognised. Advice on contraception should be offered to women of childbearing age with significant left ventricular systolic dysfunction as the haemodynamic upset of pregnancy can be poorly tolerated and maternal mortality is high. As both heart failure and the contraceptive pill increase the risk of thromboembolic disease, it may be preferable to use non-hormonal contraception, but this needs to be carefully considered on an individual basis.

Smoking

Cigarette smoking should be strongly discouraged in patients with heart failure. In addition to the well established adverse effects on coronary disease, which is the underlying cause in a substantial proportion of patients, smoking has adverse haemodynamic effects in patients with congestive heart failure. For example, smoking tends to reduce cardiac output, especially in patients with a history of myocardial infarction.

Other adverse haemodynamic effects include an increase in heart rate and systemic blood pressure (double product) and mild increases in pulmonary artery pressure, ventricular filling pressures, and total systemic and pulmonary vascular resistance.

Peripheral vasoconstriction may contribute to the observed mild reduction in stroke volume, and thus smoking increases oxygen demand and also decreases myocardial oxygen supply owing to reduced diastolic filling time (with faster heart rates) and increased carboxyhaemoglobin concentrations.

Alcohol

In general, alcohol consumption should be restricted to moderate levels, given the myocardial depressant properties of alcohol. In addition to the direct toxic effects of alcohol on the myocardium, a high alcohol intake predisposes to arrhythmias (especially atrial fibrillation) and hypertension and may lead to important alterations in fluid balance, especially with heavy beer drinking. The prognosis in alcohol-induced cardiomyopathy is poor if consumption continues, and abstinence should be advised. Abstinence can result in marked improvements, with echocardiographic studies showing substantial clinical benefit and improvements in left ventricular function.

Immunisation and antibiotic prophylaxis

Chronic heart failure predisposes to and can be exacerbated by pulmonary infection. Influenza and pneumococcal

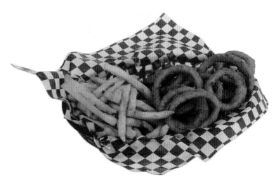

Patients should avoid foods that are rich in salt (www.photos.com)

Commonly consumed processed foods that have a high sodium content

- Cheese
- Sausages
- Crisps, salted peanuts
- Milk and white chocolate
- Tinned soup and tinned vegetables
- Ham, bacon, tinned meat (for example, corned beef)
- Tinned fish (for example, sardines, salmon, tuna)
- Smoked fish

Intrauterine devices are a suitable form of contraception, though these may be a problem in patients with primary valvar disease because of the risks of infection and risks associated with oral anticoagulation

Community and social support

- Community support is particularly important for elderly or functionally restricted patients with chronic heart failure
- Support may help to improve the quality of life and reduce admission rates
- Support from social services and community based interventions, with advice and assistance for close relatives, is also important

Date									
Pulse									
BP (lying)									
BP (standing)									
Urine									
Weight									
Drug 1									
Drug 2									
Drug 3									
Drug 4									
Drug 5									
Drug 6									
Serum urea/creatinine									
Serum potassium									
Other investigations									
Next visit									
Doctor's signature									

Heart failure cooperation card: patients and doctors are able to monitor changes in clinical signs (including weight), drug treatment, and baseline investigations. Patients should be encouraged to monitor their weight between clinic visits

vaccinations should therefore be considered in all patients with heart failure. Antibiotic prophylaxis for dental and other surgical procedures is mandatory in patients with primary valve disease and prosthetic heart valves.

Diet and nutrition

Though controlled trials offer only limited information on diet and nutritional measures, such measures are as important in heart failure as in any other chronic illness to ensure adequate and appropriate nutritional balance. Poor nutrition may contribute to cardiac cachexia, though malnutrition is not limited to patients with obvious weight loss and muscle wasting.

Patients with chronic heart failure are at an increased risk from malnutrition because of

- A decreased intake resulting from a poor appetite, which may be related to drug treatment (for example, aspirin, digoxin), metabolic disturbance (for example, hyponatraemia or renal failure), or hepatic congestion
- Malabsorption, particularly in patients with severe heart failure and
- Increased nutritional requirements, with patients with congestive heart failure having an increase of up to 20% in basal metabolic rate.

These factors may contribute to a net catabolic state in which lean muscle mass is reduced, leading to an increase in symptoms and reduced exercise capacity. Indeed, cardiac cachexia is an independent risk factor for mortality in patients with chronic heart failure. A formal nutritional assessment should thus be considered in those patients who seem to have a poor nutritional state.

Weight loss in obese patients should be encouraged as excess body mass increases cardiac workload during exercise. Obese patients should be encouraged to lose weight to within 10% of the optimal body weight.

Exercise training and rehabilitation

Exercise training benefits patients with heart failure: patients show an improvement in symptoms, a greater sense of wellbeing, and better functional capacity. Exercise does not, however, result in obvious improvement in cardiac function.

All stable patients with heart failure should be encouraged to participate in a supervised, simple exercise programme. Though bed rest ("armchair treatment") may be appropriate in patients with acute heart failure, regular exercise should be encouraged in patients with chronic heart failure. Indeed, chronic immobility may result in loss of muscle mass in the lower limb and generalised physical deconditioning, leading to a further reduction in exercise capacity and a predisposition to thromboembolism. Deconditioning itself may be detrimental, with peripheral alterations and central abnormalities leading to vasoconstriction, further deterioration in left ventricular function, and greater reduction in functional capacity.

Importantly, regular exercise has the potential to slow or stop this process and exert beneficial effects on the autonomic profile, with reduced sympathetic activity and enhanced vagal tone, thus reversing some of the adverse consequences of heart failure.

In 1999, Belardinelli published a study showing significant benefits in peak oxygen uptake, thallium scintigraphy score, and quality of life. Despite the small size of the study (99 patients), a major reduction in mortality and admission to hospital was found with exercise. The participants were relatively young (mean age 59 years), and the results of further

---

Managing cachexia in chronic heart failure

Combined management by physician and dietician is recommended
- Alter size and frequency of meals
- Ensure a higher energy diet
- Supplement diet with
  — Water soluble vitamins (loss associated with diuresis)
  — Fat soluble vitamins (levels reduced as a result of poor absorption)
  — Fish oils

Based on recommendations from the Scottish Intercollegiate Guidelines Network (SIGN) (publication No 35, 1999)

Fresh produce, such as fruit, vegetables, eggs, and fish, has a relatively low salt content

---

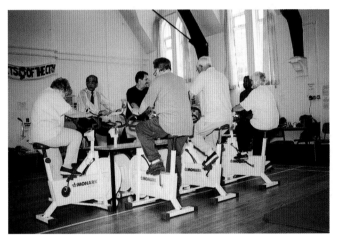

Exercise class for group of patients with heart failure. With permission of participants

---

Beneficial effects of exercise in chronic heart failure

Has positive effects on:
- Skeletal muscle
- Autonomic function
- Endothelial function
- Neurohormonal function
- Insulin sensitivity
- Quality of life measures

Effects on survival are still uncertain

studies, hopefully confirming these impressive benefits in larger and more generalisable populations, are awaited.

Regular exercise should therefore be advocated in stable patients as there is the potential for improvements in exercise tolerance and quality of life, without deleterious effects on left ventricular function. Cardiac rehabilitation services offer benefit to this group, though the exercise programme prescribed will often have to be more gentle than that for other cardiac patients, and patients should be encouraged to develop their own regular exercise routine, including walking, cycling, and swimming. Nevertheless, patients should know their limits, and excessive fatigue or breathlessness should be avoided. In the first instance, a structured walking programme would be the easiest to adopt.

Treatment of underlying disease

Treatment should also be aimed at slowing or reversing any underlying disease process.

Hypertension
Good blood pressure control is essential, and care is needed with antihypertensive drugs that have negative inotropic effects—for example, verapamil. Angiotensin converting enzyme inhibitors are the drugs of choice in patients with impaired systolic function because of their beneficial effects on slowing disease progression and improving prognosis.

In cases of isolated diastolic dysfunction, either β blockers or calcium channel blockers with rate limiting properties—for example, verapamil, diltiazem—have theoretical advantages. If severe left ventricular hypertrophy is the cause of diastolic dysfunction, however, an angiotensin converting enzyme inhibitor or angiotensin II receptor antagonist may be more effective at inducing regression of left ventricular hypertrophy.

Surgery
If coronary heart disease is the underlying cause of chronic heart failure and if cardiac ischaemia is present, the patient may benefit from coronary revascularisation, including coronary angioplasty or coronary artery bypass grafting. Revascularisation will clearly help to relieve any symptoms of angina and may also improve the function of chronically ischaemic or "hibernating" myocardium.

Valve replacement or valve repair should be considered in patients with haemodynamically important primary valve disease.

Cardiac transplantation is now established as the treatment of choice for some patients with severe heart failure who remain symptomatic despite intensive medical treatment. It is associated with a one year survival of about 85–90% and a 10 year survival of 50–60%, though it is limited by the availability of donor organs. Transplantation should be considered in younger patients (aged <60) who are without severe concomitant disease (for example, renal failure or malignancy).

This chapter was adapted from the corresponding one in the first edition written by CR Gibbs, G Jackson, and GYH Lip. Our colleagues' previous contribution is gratefully acknowledged.

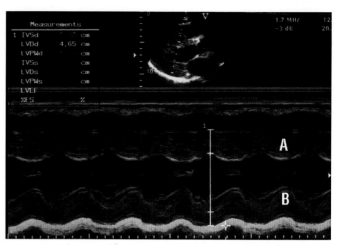

M mode echocardiogram showing left ventricular hypertrophy in hypertensive patient (A = interventricular septum; B = posterior wall of left ventricle)

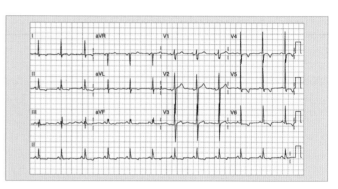

Electrocardiogram showing left ventricular hypertrophy on voltage criteria, with associated T wave and ST changes in the lateral leads ("strain pattern")

Further reading
- Belardinelli R, Georgiou D, Cianci G, Purcaro A. Randomized, controlled trial of long-term moderate exercise training in chronic heart failure: effects on functional capacity, quality of life, and clinical outcome. *Circulation* 1999; 99:1173–1182.
- Demakis JG, Proskey A, Rahimtoola SH, Jamil M, Sutton GC, Rosen KM, et al. The natural course of alcoholic cardiomyopathy. *Ann Intern Med* 1974;80:293–7.
- Task Force of the Working Group on Heart Failure of the European Society of Cardiology. Guidelines on the treatment of heart failure. *Eur Heart J* 1997;18:736–53.
- Kostis JB, Rosen RC, Cosgrove NM, Shindler DM, Wilson AC. Nonpharmacologic therapy improves functional and emotional status in congestive heart failure. *Chest* 1994;106:996–1001.
- McKelvie RS, Teo KK, McCartney N, Humen D, Montague T, Yusuf S. Effects of exercise training in patients with congestive heart failure: a critical review. *J Am Coll Cardiol* 1995;25:789–96.

7 Device therapy for heart failure

Cardiac resynchronisation therapy

In the echocardiographic heart of England screening (ECHOES) study (see chapter 1) echocardiography showed that 21% of those with a left ventricular ejection fraction <40% in the community had left bundle branch block. Over a third of those with more severe left ventricular dysfunction and more severe symptoms also had left bundle branch block.

The presence of a bundle branch block is often associated with a dyssynchronous left ventricular activation sequence, with the interventricular septum moving paradoxically when the inferoposterior wall is contracting, then contracting when the inferoposterior wall is relaxing. Thus the myocardium expends energy moving blood around the left ventricle, with a reduced amount being ejected through the aortic valve. Also, the width of the QRS complex is an important predictor of mortality in heart failure. The observation of dyssynchrony led to the concept that pacing the left ventricle via an epicardial vein, reached via the coronary sinus, at the same time as the right ventricle is paced apically, could improve this dyssynchrony, and hence biventricular pacing or cardiac resynchronisation therapy (CRT) was developed.

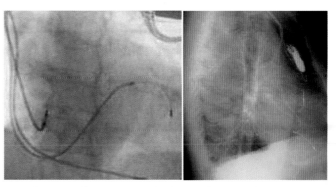

x ray of patient with cardiac resynchronisation therapy. Pacing leads are seen in the right ventricle and atrium and, via the coronary sinus, an epicaridal vein next to the left ventricle

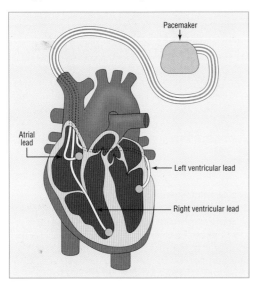

Position of leads of CRT pacemaker

Small studies proved that mechanical synchrony could be improved on echocardiography, with additional haemodynamic improvements and alleviation of the symptoms of heart failure. In the longer term, a reversal of the adverse remodelling of the heart has been observed. In addition to the effects of CRT on electrical and mechanical synchrony of the left ventricle (intraventricular synchrony), benefits have also been observed in interventricular dyssynchrony, a reduction of presystolic mitral regurgitation, and diastolic ventricular interaction. In patients with sinus rhythm, the addition of an atrial lead also allows for optimisation of the atrioventricular contraction sequence (shorter A-V conduction delay), which can further improve cardiac output in some cases.

Several large trials of CRT have now been reported, with slightly varying entry criteria in terms of QRS width on the electrocardiogram, degree of left ventricular impairment, and severity of symptoms. Impressive results have been consistently observed in terms of symptomatic improvement and reduction of

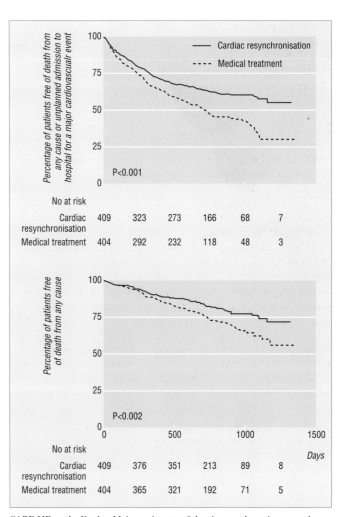

CARE-HF study: Kaplan-Meier estimates of the time to the primary end point—death from any cause or an unplanned admission to hospital for a major cardiovascular event (top) and the principal secondary outcome—death from any cause (bottom). Adapted from Cleland J, et al. *N Engl J Med* 2005;352:877–83

ABC of heart failure

hospital admission rates. A trend toward reduction of mortality was observed, and a clear reduction in mortality was first reported in the recent CARE-HF (cardiac resynchronization-heart failure) study. This study showed a 37% reduction in all cause mortality or unplanned cardiovascular admission to hospital over 29.4 months associated with CRT. It improved all cause mortality, echocardiographic indices, and symptoms and quality of life.

The results of the CARE-HF study (with other studies of CRT) are likely to lead to considerable increases in implantation of these devices in the coming years. Some patients, however, do not seem to respond to treatment as well as others and some further refinement of implantation criteria is likely. Some patients have shown dyssynchrony even in the absence of left bundle branch block, and they may also benefit from CRT.

Implantable cardioverter defibrillators

Many studies have shown that the mode of death in patients with heart failure is evenly split between progressive heart failure and sudden unexpected events. These sudden events have often been assumed to be due to fatal ventricular arrhythmias, but postmortem studies have suggested that new coronary occlusive events are also important.

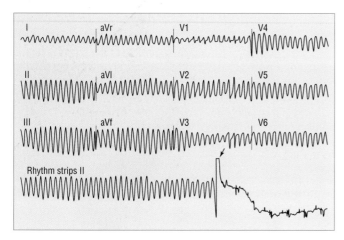

Patient with a malignant ventricular arrhythmia terminated by shock from an implantable cardioverter defibrillator (arrow)

The advent of implantable cardioverter defibrillators (ICDs), their safe implantation via a transvenous route, and the proof of their effectiveness in saving lives in patients with cardiac dysfunction and known ventricular arrhythmias has led to trials of prophylactic ICD therapy in those with cardiac dysfunction and heart failure but no previously documented arrhythmias.

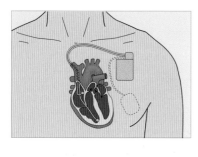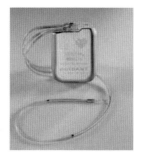

Implantable cardioverter defibrillator

Over 20 months the Multicenter automatic defibrillator implantation trial-II (MADIT-II) showed a 31% reduction in all cause mortality in those receiving an ICD. All patients had previous myocardial infarction and left ventricular ejection fraction of <30%.

Entry criteria for CARE-HF*

- Age >18 years of age
- Heart failure for at least six weeks
- New York Heart Association (NYHA) class III or IV despite receipt of standard pharmacological therapy
- Left ventricular ejection fraction <35%; a left ventricular end diastolic dimension of ≥30 mm (indexed to height)
- QRS interval of ≥120 msec on the electrocardiogram*

*Patients with a QRS interval of 120–149 msec had to meet two of three additional criteria for dyssynchrony: an aortic pre-ejection delay of >140 msec, an interventricular mechanical delay of >40 msec, or delayed activation of the posterolateral left ventricular wall.
Patients who had had a major cardiovascular event in the previous six weeks, those who had conventional indications for a pacemaker or an implantable defibrillator, and those with heart failure requiring continuous intravenous therapy were excluded. Also excluded were patients with atrial arrhythmias, as such patients could not benefit from the atrial component of resynchronisation.

*Adapted from Cleland J, et al. *N Engl J Med* 2005;352:877-83

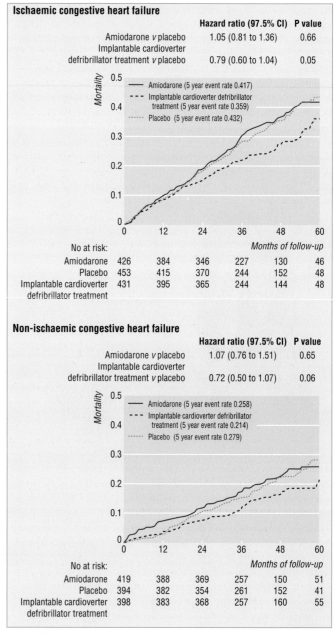

Kaplan-Meier estimates of death from any cause for the prespecified subgroups of ischaemic congestive heart failure (top) and non-ischaemic congestive heart failure (bottom). Adapted from Bardy G, et al. *N Engl J Med* 2005;352:225-37

Subsequently, the sudden cardiac death in heart failure trial (SCD-HeFT) showed the benefits of prophylactic ICD use in a wider population with NYHA class II and III heart failure and left ventricular ejection fraction of <35%, of either ischaemic or idiopathic origin (that is, dilated cardiomyopathy). They also showed a 23% reduction in all cause mortality compared with amiodarone or placebo over nearly four years. Amiodarone, disappointingly, had no favourable effect on survival, and the benefit of ICD therapy was found in patients with ischaemic and idiopathic heart failure. All of the mortality benefit, however, was seen in those with milder (NYHA class II) symptoms. Although this may have been a chance finding on subgroup analysis, it does suggest that those with more severe symptoms may be more likely to die of progressive heart failure and less likely to benefit from a prophylactic ICD.

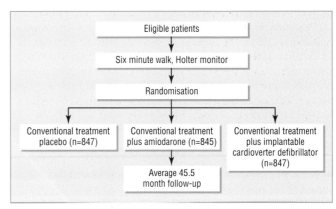

Details of the sudden cardiac death in heart failure trial. Adapted from Bardy G, et al. *N Engl J Med* 2005;352:225–37

Combined cardiac resynchronisation and defibrillators

It is apparent that patients with heart failure who are candidates for CRT will also meet the MADIT-II study entry criteria and may therefore benefit from implantation of a combined CRT and ICD device, sometimes referred to as "high energy CRT," as they are also at risk of arrhythmias and sudden death. The evidence for CRT, however, is largely confined to those with NYHA class III and IV symptoms, and subgroup analysis of the MADIT-II study suggested that such patients derived less survival benefit than those with NYHA class II symptoms.

The question of which device was preferable was examined in the comparison of medical therapy, pacing, and defibrillation in heart failure (COMPANION) study. In this, patients with NYHA class III or IV heart failure, left ventricular ejection fraction <35% (ischaemic and non-ischaemic aetiology), and QRS width >120 ms were randomised on a 1:2:2 basis to receive optimal medical therapy alone or with CRT or a CRT/defibrillator. The 12 month death rate from any cause or rate of admission to

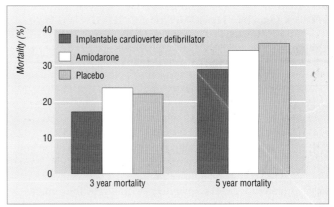

Mortality results from SCD-HeFT. Adapted from Bardy G, et al. *N Engl J Med* 2005;352:225–37.

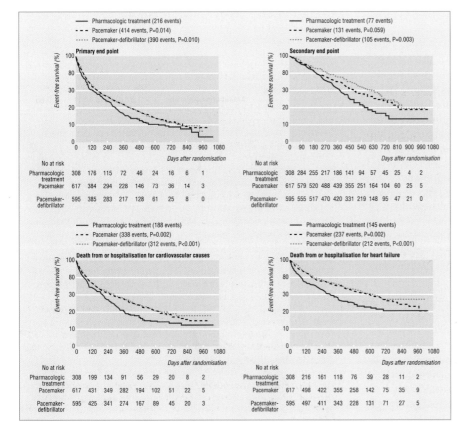

Main results from the COMPANION study of medical therapy, CRT, and CRT-Defibrillator. The top left graph shows time to the primary end point of death from or hospitalisation for any cause. The top right graph shows time to the secondary end point of death from any cause. The bottom left graph shows time to death from or hospitalisation for cardiovascular causes, and the bottom right graph shows time to death from or hospitalisation for heart failure. Adapted from Bristow MR, et al. *N Engl J Med* 2004;350:2140–50

hospital for any cause was 68% in the medical therapy group and 56% in both the CRT and CRT/defibrillator groups (significant reductions of about 20% in both). The secondary end point of all cause mortality was 19% in the medical therapy group; it was 24% lower in the CRT group (just failing to reach significance) but 36% lower in the CRT/defibrillator group (P = 0.004). Both device therapy groups derived measurable additional benefits in symptoms, quality of life, and blood pressure.

Who should get which device?

Both CRT and ICD treatments are clearly highly effective clinically, but both are expensive and there are large numbers of potential candidates for treatment. This has led to much debate regarding the cost effectiveness of treatment and which device to use in which setting. Further research findings, and also possible reductions in the price of the devices, are likely to influence conclusions in the future.

Invasive haemodynamic monitoring

The implantable haemodynamic monitor (Chronicle, Medtronic) has been designed to continuously monitor intracardiac pressure, body temperature, physical activity, and heart rate in patients with systolic and diastolic heart failure (NYHA class III and IV). In the Chronicle offers management to patients with advances signs and symptoms of heart failure (COMPASS-HF) study, the use of the device led to a 33% reduction in patients experiencing worsening heart failure and fewer emergency assessments and admissions to hospital. It is not clear whether similar benefits could have been gained from simple non-invasive measurements carried out by the patients themselves (weight, pulse, and blood pressure with an automated device) and frequent telephone contact with a specialist nurse. Measurement of thoracic impedance via a pacemaker and its lead can also be used to estimate pulmonary congestion.

Left ventricular assist devices

Heart transplantation will always be a treatment for only a small minority of those with end stage heart failure because of the limited number of donor organs available. Prototypes of total artificial hearts have been unsuccessful owing to thrombosis, haemolysis, the need for an external power source, infection, etc. Left ventricular assist devices, which pump blood from the left ventricular cavity into the aorta, thereby easing the work for the native heart and working in parallel with the heart, are now well established as a "bridge" to transplantation, and research is now taking place into their possible role as "destination" therapy. Tunnelled leads, with a power pedestal emerging on the scalp via the skull, seem to be a solution to the problem of the power supply and lead infection, and event-free survival up to four years has been reported, with improved quality of life. Randomised trials comparing such treatment with optimal medical therapy (and established device therapy) are needed.

Other non-invasive mechanical devices

External counterpulsation, using intermittent inflation of large "trousers," has been used to improve exercise tolerance in some patients with heart failure, but long term improvements have not been shown as yet. Continuous positive airways pressure is useful if there is concomitant obstructive sleep apnoea with heart failure but has not proved to be of benefit in cases of central sleep apnoea, which is common in patients with heart failure.

Which device?

- All patients should be titrated up to maximum tolerated or evidence based maximum medical therapy
- Those with persistent NYHA class III and IV symptoms, ejection fraction <35%, QRS duration of >120 ms, and demonstration of dyssynchrony if the QRS duration is 120–149 ms, should be considered for CRT. The additional benefit of defibrillation function is likely to be fairly limited and costly, so CRT/defibrillators may be best reserved for those with indication for CRT and 'conventional' indication for an ICD—that is, documented ventricular arrhythmias
- Those with ejection fraction <30% after myocardial infarction, and those with NYHA class II symptoms and ejection fraction <35%, irrespective of aetiology and QRS duration, should be considered for prophylactic ICD implantation on the basis of the MADIT-II and SCD HeFT results. Healthcare purchasers need to examine the issues of cost effectiveness and affordability of such treatment

---

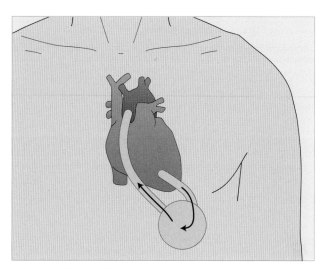

Left ventricular assist device

Further reading

- Bardy GH, Lee KL, Mark DB, Poole JE, Packer DL, Boineau R, et al. Sudden cardiac death in heart failure trial (SCD-HeFT) investigators. Amiodarone or an implantable cardioverter-defibrillator for congestive heart failure. *N Engl J Med* 2005;352:225–37.
- Bristow MR, Saxon LA, Boehmer J, Krueger S, Kass DA, De Marco T, et al. Comparison of medical therapy, pacing, and defibrillation in heart failure (COMPANION) investigators. Cardiac-resynchronization therapy with or without an implantable defibrillator in advanced chronic heart failure. *N Engl J Med* 2004;350:2140–50.
- Cleland JG, Daubert JC, Erdmann E, Freemantle N, Gras D, Kappenberger L, et al. Cardiac resynchronization-heart failure (CARE-HF) study investigators. The effect of cardiac resynchronization on morbidity and mortality in heart failure. *N Engl J Med* 2005;352:1539–49.
- Moss AJ, Zareba W, Hall WJ, Klein H, Wilber DJ, Cannom DS, et al. Multicenter automatic defibrillator implantation trial II investigators. Prophylactic implantation of a defibrillator in patients with myocardial infarction and reduced ejection fraction. *N Engl J Med* 2002;346:877–83.
- Siegenthaler MP, Westaby S, Frazier OH, Martin J, Banning A, Robson D, et al. Advanced heart failure: feasibility study of long-term continuous axial flow pump support. *Eur Heart J* 2005;26:1031–8.

8 Management: diuretics, ACE inhibitors, and angiotensin receptor antagonists, and vasodilators

In the past 20 years several large scale randomised controlled trials have revolutionised the management of patients with chronic heart failure. Though it is clear that some drugs improve symptoms, others offer both symptomatic and prognostic benefits, and the management of heart failure should be aimed at improving both quality of life and survival.

Diuretics, angiotensin converting enzyme (ACE) inhibitors, and β blockers, when combined with non-pharmacological measures, are now accepted as standard treatment in patients with congestive heart failure. Angiotensin receptor blockers are now established as alternatives to ACE inhibitors in those with intolerance and can also have a role in combination with ACE inhibitors. Aldosterone antagonism is valuable in selected cases, though care needs to be used in patient monitoring. Digoxin still has a possible role in some of these patients, though there is no evidence that it improves survival.

Diuretics

Diuretics are effective in providing symptomatic relief and remain the first line treatment, particularly in the presence of oedema. Nevertheless, there is no direct evidence that loop and thiazide diuretics confer prognostic benefit in patients with congestive heart failure.

Loop diuretics

Loop diuretics—such as furosemide (frusemide), bumetanide, and torasemide—have a powerful diuretic action, increasing the excretion of sodium and water via their action on the ascending limb of the loop of Henle. They have a rapid onset of action (five minutes intravenously, one to two hours orally; duration of action four to six hours). Oral absorption of furosemide may be reduced in congestive heart failure, and the pharmacokinetics of bumetanide and torasemide may allow improved bioavailability in this setting.

Patients receiving high dose diuretics (frusemide ≥80 mg or equivalent) should be monitored for renal and electrolyte abnormalities. Hypokalaemia, which may precipitate arrhythmias, should be avoided, though this is much less common than previously since ACE inhibitors and aldosterone antagonists have become standard treatment, and potassium supplementation is now only occasionally needed. Acute gout is a relatively common adverse effect of treatment with high dose diuretics.

Thiazide diuretics

Thiazides—such as bendroflumethiazide (bendrofluazide)—act on the cortical diluting segment of the nephron. They are often ineffective in elderly people because of the reduction in glomerular filtration rate associated with age and heart failure. Hyponatraemia and hypokalaemia are commonly associated with higher doses of thiazide diuretics, and potassium supplementation, or concomitant treatment with a potassium sparing agent, is usually needed with high dose thiazide therapy. For these reasons, thiazides are not normally used as first line agents to control fluid status in heart failure. In milder cases, they can prove useful in controlling blood pressure.

Aims of heart failure management

To achieve improvement in symptoms
- Diuretics
- Digoxin
- ACE inhibitors/angiotensin receptor blockers

To achieve improvement in survival
- ACE inhibitors/angiotensin receptor blockers
- β blockers (for example, carvedilol and bisoprolol)
- Oral nitrates plus hydralazine
- Spironolactone

In general, diuretics should be introduced at a low dose and the dose increased according to the clinical response. There are dangers, however, in either undertreating or overtreating patients with diuretics, and regular review is necessary

---

How to use diuretics in patients with advanced heart failure
- Use the minimum diuretic dose required to control fluid status
- Combination diuretic treatment with a loop diuretic and aldosterone antagonist may improve survival as well as symptoms, but caution is needed due to risk of hyperkalaemia when used with an ACE inhibitor
- Administer loop diuretics intravenously if response to oral therapy is inadequate—infusion may provide a smoother and better tolerated effect than large boluses
- Thiazide or thiazide-like diuretics may be useful in addition to loop diuretics in resistant cases. Careful monitoring of renal function is necessary

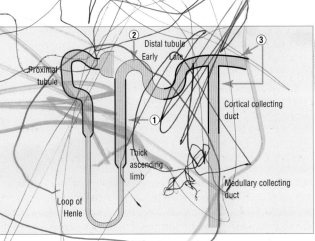

Diagram of nephron showing sites of action of different diuretic classes: 1=loop (for example, furosemide); 2=thiazide (for example, bendroflumethiazide); and 3=potassium sparing (for example, amiloride)

ABC of heart failure

In some patients with chronic severe congestive heart failure, particularly in the presence of chronic renal impairment, oedema may persist despite conventional oral doses (furosemide 40–160 mg daily) of loop diuretics. In these patients, a thiazide diuretic (for example, bendroflumethazide) or a thiazide-like diuretic (for example, metolazone) may be combined with a loop diuretic. This combination blocks reabsorption of sodium at different sites in the nephron ("double nephron blockade"), and this synergistic action leads to a greater diuretic effect. The incidence of associated metabolic abnormalities is, however, increased, and such treatment should be started only under close supervision. In some patients, a large diuretic effect may occur soon after a combination regimen (loop diuretic plus either thiazide or metalozone) has been started. It is advisable, therefore, to consider such a combination treatment on a twice weekly basis, at least initially.

Potassium sparing diuretics

Amiloride acts on the distal nephron, while spironolactone is a competitive aldosterone antagonist. Potassium sparing diuretics need to be used with caution in patients receiving ACE inhibitors because of the potential risk of hyperkalaemia. In patients with heart failure treated with ACE inhibitors, aldosterone concentrations commonly rise as the disease progresses, after falling when the ACE inhibitor was started ("aldosterone escape"). The rise in aldosterone can cause further deleterious effects—for example, myocardial fibrosis and remodelling. The randomised spironolactone (Aldactone) evaluation study (RALES) showed a major survival benefit associated with the use of spironolactone in addition to background therapy including ACE inhibitors. The risk of hyperkalaemia seemed to be low when low dose spironolactone (25 mg daily) was combined with an ACE inhibitor. Many in the UK have found more of a problem with the development of hyperkalaemia, possibly because the study entry criteria of a baseline potassium concentrations of <5.0 mmol/l and creatinine of <223 μmol/l are not adhered to. Serum creatinine and potassium concentrations should be measured five to seven days after the addition of a potassium sparing diuretic to an ACE inhibitor until the concentrations are stable and then every one to three months. The American Heart Association/American College of Cardiology have issued guidelines for minimising the risk of hyperkalaemia in patients treated with aldosterone.

Eplerenone may be an effective alternative in patients who cannot tolerate spironolactone (particularly if side effects of feminisation predominate) but is not licensed for chronic heart failure but for heart failure in the early stages after a myocardial infarction.

ACE inhibitors

ACE inhibitors have consistently shown beneficial effects on mortality, morbidity, and quality of life in large scale prospective clinical trials and are indicated in all stages of symptomatic heart failure resulting from impaired left ventricular systolic function. These agents are also useful in asymptomatic heart failure to slow rate of progression.

Mechanisms of action

ACE inhibitors inhibit the enzyme converting angiotensin I to angiotensin II, which is a potent vasoconstrictor and growth promoter. Angiotensin II also causes the release of aldosterone by the adrenal cortex, and this has deleterious effects in the long term in heart failure. ACE inhibitors also increase concentrations of the vasodilator bradykinin by inhibiting its degradation via the enzyme chymase. Bradykinin has been shown to have beneficial

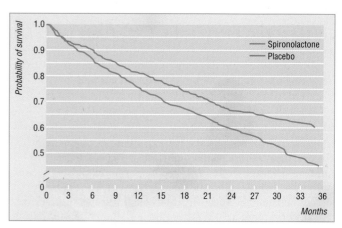

Survival curve for randomised spironolactone (Aldactone) evaluation study (RALES) showing 30% reduction in all cause mortality when spironolactone (up to 25 mg) was added to conventional treatment in patients with severe (NYHA class IV) chronic heart failure

---

Guidelines for minimising the risk of hyperkalaemia in patients treated with aldosterone antagonists (American Heart Association/American College of Cardiology)

- Impaired renal function is a risk factor for hyperkalaemia during treatment with aldosterone antagonists. The risk of hyperkalaemia increases progressively when serum creatinine >122 μmol/l. In elderly patients or others with low muscle mass in whom serum creatinine concentration does not accurately reflect glomerular filtration rate, determination that glomerular filtration rate or creatinine clearance >0.50 ml/s is recommended
- Aldosterone antagonists should not be administered to patients with baseline serum potassium >5.0 mmol/l
- An initial dose of 12.5 mg spironolactone or 25 mg eplerenone is recommended, after which the dose may be increased to 25 mg spironolactone or 50 mg eplerenone if appropriate
- The risk of hyperkalaemia is increased with concomitant use of higher doses of ACE inhibitors (captopril ≥75 mg daily; enalapril or lisinopril ≥10 mg daily).
- Non-steroidal anti-inflammatory drugs and cyclo-oxygenase 2 inhibitors should be avoided
- Potassium supplements should be discontinued or reduced
- Close monitoring of serum potassium is required; potassium concentrations and renal function should be checked in three days and at one week after initiation of therapy and at least monthly for the first three months
- Diarrhoea or other causes of dehydration should be addressed emergently

---

Guidelines for using ACE inhibitors

- Stop potassium supplements and potassium sparing diuretics
- Omit (or reduce) diuretics for 24 hours before first close
- Advise patient to sit or lie down for two to four hours after the first dose
- Start low doses (for example, captopril 6.25 mg twice daily, enalapril 2.5 mg once daily, lisinopril 2.5 mg once daily)
- Review after one to two weeks to reassess symptoms, blood pressure, and renal chemistry and electrolytes
- Increase dose unless there has been a rise in serum creatinine concentration (to >200 μmol/l) or potassium concentration (to >5.0 mmol/l)
- Titrate to maximum tolerated dose, reassessing blood pressure and renal chemistry and electrolytes after each dose titration

If patient is "high risk" consider hospital admission to start treatment

effects associated with the release of nitric oxide and prostacyclin, which may contribute to the positive haemodynamic effects of the ACE inhibitors. Bradykinin may also be responsible, however, for some of the adverse effects, such as dry cough, hypotension, and angio-oedema.

ACE inhibitors also reduce the activity of the sympathetic nervous system as angiotensin II promotes the release of noradrenaline (norepinephrine) and inhibits its reuptake. In addition, they also improve β receptor density (causing their up regulation), variation in heart rate, baroreceptor function, and autonomic function (including vagal tone).

Clinical effects
Symptomatic left ventricular dysfunction
ACE inhibitors improve symptoms, exercise tolerance, and survival and reduce hospital admission rates in chronic heart failure.

These beneficial effects are apparent in all grades of systolic heart failure—that is, mild to moderate chronic heart failure (as evident, for example, in the Munich mild heart failure study, the vasodilator heart failure trials (V-HeFT), and the studies of left ventricular dysfunction treatment trial (SOLVD-T)) and severe chronic heart failure (as, for example, in the first cooperative north Scandinavian enalapril survival study (CONSENSUS I).

Asymptomatic left ventricular dysfunction
ACE inhibitors have also been shown to be effective in asymptomatic patients with left ventricular systolic dysfunction. The studies of left ventricular dysfunction prevention trial (SOLVD-P) confirmed the benefit of ACE inhibitors in asymptomatic left ventricular systolic dysfunction, where enalapril reduced the development of heart failure and related hospital admissions.

Left ventricular dysfunction after myocardial infarction
Large scale randomised controlled trials—for example, the acute infarction ramipril efficacy (AIRE) study, the survival and ventricular enlargement (SAVE) study, and the trial of trandolapril cardiac evaluation (TRACE)—have shown lower mortality in patients with impaired systolic function after myocardial infarction, irrespective of symptoms.

Slowing disease progression
ACE inhibitors also seem to influence the natural course of chronic heart failure. The Munich mild heart failure study showed that ACE inhibitors combined with standard treatment slowed the progression of heart failure in patients with mild symptoms, with significantly fewer patients in the active treatment group developing severe heart failure.

Doses and tolerability
ACE inhibitors should be started at a low dose and gradually titrated to the highest tolerated maintenance level. The (recent) prospective assessment trial of lisinopril and survival (ATLAS) randomised patients with symptomatic heart failure to low dose (2.5 − 5.0 mg daily) or high dose (32.5 − 35.0 mg daily) lisinopril, and, though there was no significant difference in mortality, high dose treatment was associated with a significant reduction in the combined end point of all cause mortality and all cause admissions to hospital. Adverse effects of the ACE inhibitors include cough, dizziness, and deterioration in renal function, though the overall incidence of hypotension and renal impairment in the CONSENSUS and SOLVD studies was only 5%. Angio-oedema related to ACE inhibitors is rare, though more common in patients of Afro-Caribbean origin than in other ethnic groups.

ACE inhibitors can therefore be regarded as the cornerstone of treatment in patients with all grades of symptomatic heart

---

High risk patients who warrant close observation when starting ACE inhibitors

- Severe heart failure (New York Heart Association (NYHA) class IV) or decompensated heart failure
- Low systolic blood pressure (<100 mm Hg)
- Resting tachycardia >100 beats/minute
- Low serum sodium concentration (<130 mmol/1)
- Other vasodilator treatment
- Severe chronic obstructive airways disease and pulmonary heart disease (cor pulmonale)

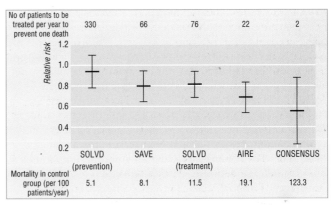

ACE inhibitors in left ventricular dysfunction: best benefit for ACE inhibitors in higher risk group. Adapted with permission from Smith D, et al. *BMJ* 1994;308:73–4

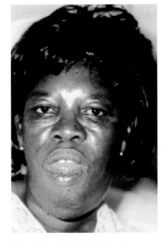
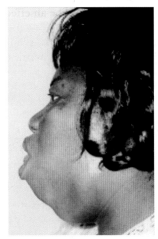

Front view and side view of a woman with angio-oedema related to treatment with ACE inhibitors. Published with permission of patient

failure and in patients with asymptomatic left ventricular dysfunction. Every attempt should be made to provide this treatment for patients, unless it is contraindicated, and to use adequate doses.

Angiotensin receptor antagonists

Orally active angiotensin II type 1 receptor antagonists, such as candesartan, losartan, and valsartan, represent a new class of agents that offer an alternative method of blocking the renin-angiotensin system. The effects of angiotensin II receptor antagonists on haemodynamics, neuroendocrine activity, and exercise tolerance resemble those of ACE inhibitors.

The evaluation of losartan in the elderly II (ELITE II) study failed to show that treatment with losartan was superior to captopril, though losartan was better tolerated. It is possible that the losartan dose was too low in this study (50 mg per day). The more recent candesartan in heart failure: assessment of reduction in mortality and morbidity-alternative (CHARM-alternative) trial compared candesartan with placebo in patients with chronic systolic heart failure and documented intolerance to ACE inhibitors and found unequivocal evidence of benefit.

One study, the CHARM-added trial, has showed benefit of using candesartan in addition to ACE inhibitors in patients with systolic heart failure. Both cardiovascular mortality and hospital admission were significantly reduced, and these benefits were seen despite all participants receiving ACE inhibitors, 55% receiving β blockers, and 17% receiving spironolactone at baseline.

Valsartan has been shown to be as good as an ACE inhibitor in reducing cardiovascular end points after myocardial infarction. A combination of valsartan and captopril did not have a significant additive beneficial effect but resulted in more side effects.

Oral nitrates and hydralazine

The first treatment shown to improve prognosis in heart failure was not ACE inhibition but the combined use of vasodilators in the form of the nitric oxide donor, isosorbide dinitrate, and hydralazine, an antihypertensive with antioxidant properties. The use of this combination fell as the evidence for ACE inhibitors grew, and a subsequent comparison showed a greater benefit with use of the ACE inhibitor, enalapril, than the hydralazine-isosorbide dinitrate combination. The concomitant use of both an ACE inhibitor and hydralazine-isosorbide dinitrate has not been studied until recently. In view of the differential response to the drugs in different races, African-Americans were studied in the recent African-American heart failure trial (A-HeFT). Participants with NYHA class III and IV heart failure who were already taking standard therapy including an ACE inhibitor and β blocker in most cases, were randomised to receive hydralazine-isosorbide dinitrate or placebo. The study was terminated early due to a significantly higher mortality in the placebo group (10.2% v 6.2%). Admission to hospital for heart failure was also reduced in the hydralazine-isosorbide dinitrate group, and quality of life scores improved more.

The important results in a racial group thought particularly likely to benefit from this treatment have led to considerable debate about whether the results should be applied to those from other racial groups. In the US, a race specific licence has been granted for a hydralazine-isosorbide combination pill. Clearly, the trial should be repeated in other racial groups to

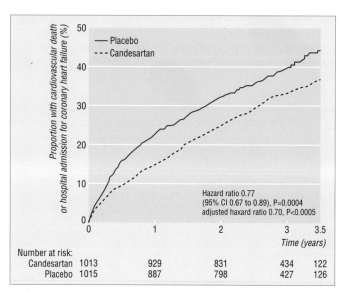

Kaplan-Meier cumulative event curves for primary outcome of the CHARM-alternative trial. Adapted from Granger C, et al. *Lancet* 2003;362:772–6

> In view of the greater weight of evidence in their favour, as well as their lower cost, ACE inhibitors currently remain the treatment of choice in patients with left ventricular systolic dysfunction, and angiotensin II receptor antagonists are an appropriate alternative in patients who develop important side effects from ACE inhibitors

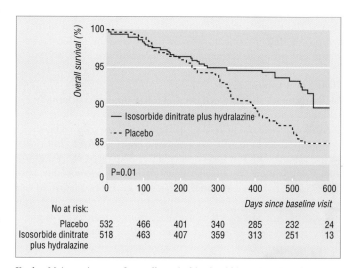

Kaplan-Meier estimates of overall survival in the African-American heart failure trial. Adapted from Taylor AL, et al. *N Engl J Med* 2004;351:2049–57

establish whether the benefits apply to them also. South Asians and other minority ethnic groups, however, have been little studied in therapeutic studies of many conditions, yet most drugs are licensed to be used in all ethnic groups. It therefore seems that, pending firm data to the contrary, those from racial groups that have not been studied should not be denied treatments shown to benefit another ethnic group.

Particularly in view of these recent data on the efficacy of hydralazine-isosorbide, the combination should certainly be considered for those unable to tolerate ACE inhibitors or angiotensin II receptor antagonists—for example, due to renal failure.

Other vasodilators

Long acting dihydropyridine calcium channel blockers generally have neutral effects in heart failure, though others, such as diltiazem and verapamil, have negatively inotropic and chronotropic properties, with the potential to exacerbate heart failure. The prospective randomised amlodipine survival evaluation (PRAISE) study showed the safety of the dihydropyridine, amlodipine, in patients with congestive heart failure, though no extra benefit for heart failure was seen. Similar observations were seen for felodipine in the V-HeFT III trial. Thus, amlodipine and felodipine, which are both long acting dihydropyridine calcium antagonists, can be useful drugs to treat angina and hypertension in this group of patients.

This chapter was adapted from the corresponding one in the first edition written by MK Davies, CR Gibbs, and GYH Lip. Our colleague's previous contribution is gratefully acknowledged.

Further reading

- CONSENSUS Trial Study Group. Effects of enalapril on mortality in severe congestive heart failure: results of the cooperative north Scandinavian enalapril survival study (CONSENSUS). *N Engl J Med* 1987;316:1429–35.
- Granger CB, McMurray JJ, Yusuf S, Held P, Michelson EL, et al. Effects of candesartan in patients with chronic heart failure and reduced left-ventricular systolic function intolerant to angiotensin-converting-enzyme inhibitors: the CHARM-Alternative trial. *Lancet* 2003;362:772–6.
- McMurray JJ, Ostergren J, Swedberg K, Granger CB, Michelson EL, et al. Effects of candesartan in patients with chronic heart failure and reduced left-ventricular systolic function taking angiotensin-converting-enzyme inhibitors: the CHARM-Added trial. *Lancet* 2003;362:767–71.
- Pitt B, Remme W, Zannand F, Neaton J, Martinez F, et al. Eplerenone, a selective aldosterone blocker, in patients with left ventricular dysfunction after myocardial infarction. *N Engl J Med* 2003;348:1309–21.
- Pitt B, Zannad F, Remme WJ, Cody R, Castaigne A, Perez A, et al. The effect of spironolactone on morbidity and mortality in patients with severe heart failure. *N Engl J Med* 1999;341:709–17.
- Taylor AL, Ziesche S, Yancy C, Carson P, D'Agostino R, et al. Combination of isosorbide dinitrate and hydralazine in blacks with heart failure. *N Engl J Med* 2004;351:2049–57.

9 Management: β blockers, digoxin, and other inotropes, and antiarrhythmic and antithrombotic treatment

> **Potential mechanisms and benefits of β blockers are improved left ventricular function; reduced sympathetic tone; improved autonomic nervous system balance; up regulation of β adrenergic receptors; reduction in arrhythmias, ischaemia, further infarction, myocardial fibrosis, and apoptosis**

β blockers

Traditionally it was thought that β adrenoceptor blockers were best avoided in patients with heart failure because of their negative inotropic effects. Though they may be detrimental for patients with severe decompensated heart failure, however, there is evidence that, when used carefully, they reduce the adverse effects of the chronic sympathetic overload that occurs in heart failure and that leads to further deterioration. There is now unequivocal evidence from clinical trials to support the use of β blockers in patients with chronic stable heart failure resulting from left ventricular systolic dysfunction. Many randomised controlled trials in patients with chronic heart failure have reported that combining β blockers with conventional treatment such as diuretics and angiotensin converting enzyme (ACE) inhibitors results in improvements in left ventricular function, symptoms, and survival, as well as a reduction in admissions to hospital.

Several randomised controlled trials have studied the effects of carvedilol, a β blocker with α blocking and vasodilator properties, in patients with symptomatic heart failure. The US multicentre carvedilol study programme was stopped early because of a highly significant (65%) mortality benefit in patients receiving carvedilol compared with placebo, and the Australia/New Zealand heart failure study reported a 41% reduction in the combined primary end point of all cause hospital admission and mortality. Subsequently, the carvedilol prospective randomized cumulative survival (COPERNICUS) study showed major benefits of carvedilol therapy on survival, admission to hospital, and quality of life even in those with more severe (NYHA class III and IV) heart failure.

The large cardiac insufficiency bisoprolol study II (CIBIS II), which looked at the β blocker, bisoprolol, was stopped prematurely because of the beneficial effects of active treatment on both morbidity and mortality. Metoprolol in slow release formulation (unavailable in the UK) also showed similar prognostic advantages in the metoprolol randomised intervention trial in heart failure (MERIT-HF), which was also stopped early. In 2004, the study of effects of nebivolol intervention on outcomes and rehospitalisation in seniors with heart failure (SENIORS) study also showed benefit of nebivolol, a β blocker with nitrate-like properties, in a much older (and therefore more representative of most patients in clinical practice) cohort of patients with heart failure. All of these studies compared treatment with β blocker and placebo in patients already treated with ACE inhibitors.

The CIBIS III trial found no significant difference in beneficial effects if either ACE inhibitors or β blockers were started first.

Treatment with β blockers

Who should receive β blocker therapy
- All patients with chronic, stable heart failure
- Those without contraindications (symptomatic hypotension or bradycardia, asthma)

What to tell patients
- Treatment is primarily prophylactic against death and new admissions to hospital for cardiovascular reasons
- Some patients will experience improvement of symptoms

When to start
- No physical evidence of fluid retention (use diuretics accordingly)
- Start ACE inhibitors first if not contraindicated
- In stable patients, in the hospital or in outpatient clinics
- Patients with New York Heart Association (NYHA) class IV or severe congestive heart failure should be referred for specialist advice
- Review treatment. Avoid verapamil, diltiazem, antiarrhythmics, non-steroidal anti-inflammatory drugs

β blocker
- Start with a low dose
- Increase dose slowly; double dose at not less than every two weeks
- Aim for target dose (see above) or, if not tolerated, the highest tolerated dose

Monitoring
- Monitor for evidence of symptoms of heart failure, fluid retention, hypotension, and bradycardia
- Instruct patients to weigh themselves daily and to increase their dose of diuretic if their weight increases

Adapted from European Society of Cardiology guidelines (2005)

β blockers with evidence for use in heart failure

- Carvedilol
- Metoprolol slow release
- Bisoprolol
- Nebivolol

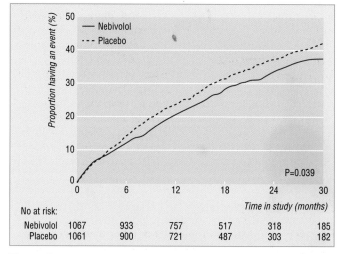

Time to first occurrence of events (all cause death or hospital admission for a cardiovascular reason—the primary endpoint) in the SENIORS trial of nebivolol in elderly patients with heart failure. Adapted from Flather MD, et al. *Eur Heart J* 2005;26:215–25

There is increasing evidence that not all β blockers are the same; bucindolol did not show significant benefit in the beta blocker evaluation of survival trial (BEST), and the carvedilol or metoprolol European trial (COMET), comparing carvedilol with normal release metoprolol, showed a significant benefit for carvedilol, with 17% lower mortality in patients with mild and moderate heart failure.

In general, β blockers should be started at very low doses, with the dose being slowly increased, under expert supervision, to the target dose if tolerated. In the short term there may be a deterioration in symptoms, which may improve with alterations in other treatment, particularly diuretics.

Digoxin

> Digoxin should be considered in patients with sinus rhythm plus *(a)* continued symptoms of heart failure despite optimal doses of diuretics and angiotensin converting enzyme inhibitors; *(b)* severe left ventricular systolic dysfunction with cardiac dilatation; or *(c)* recurrent hospital admissions for heart failure

Use of digoxin for heart failure varies between countries across Europe, with high rates in Germany and low rates in the UK. It is potentially invaluable in patients with atrial fibrillation and coexistent heart failure, improving control of the ventricular rate and allowing more effective filling of the ventricle. Digoxin is also used in patients with chronic heart failure secondary to left ventricular systolic impairment, in sinus rhythm, who remain symptomatic despite optimal doses of diuretics and angiotensin converting enzyme inhibitors, in whom it acts as an inotrope.

Symptomatic benefit from digoxin in patients with chronic heart failure in sinus rhythm has been reported in several randomised placebo controlled trials and several smaller trials. The randomised assessment of the effect of digoxin on inhibitors of the angiotensin converting enzyme (RADIANCE) and prospective randomized study of ventricular function and efficacy of digoxin (PROVED) trials, for example, reported that the withdrawal of digoxin from patients with congestive heart failure who had already been treated with the drug was associated with worsening heart failure and increased rates of readmission to hospital. The Digitalis Investigation Group's large study found that digoxin was associated with a symptomatic improvement in patients with congestive heart failure when it was added to treatment with diuretics and ACE inhibitors. Importantly, there were greater absolute and relative benefits in the patients who had resistant symptoms and more severe impairment of left ventricular systolic function. Though there was a reduction in admission and mortality resulting from heart failure, however, there was no significant improvement in overall survival. β blockers were used rarely in the study, and it is therefore not clear whether the effect of digoxin is additive to both β blockers and ACE inhibitors in congestive heart failure.

Digoxin is also best avoided immediately after myocardial infarction as higher mortality has been reported in this context.

Other inotropes

The potential role of inotropic agents, other than digoxin, in chronic heart failure has been examined in several studies. Althoughthese drugs seem to improve symptoms in some patients, most have been associated with an increase in mortality.

Problem solving in patients taking β blockers
- Reduce/discontinue β blocker only if other actions were ineffective to control symptoms/secondary effects
- Always consider the reintroduction and/or up titration of the β blocker when the patient becomes stable
- Seek specialist advice if in doubt

Symptomatic hypotension (dizziness, light headedness and/or confusion)
- Reconsider the need for nitrates, calcium channel blockers, and other vasodilators
- If no signs/symptoms of congestion consider reducing diuretic dose

Worsening symptoms/signs (increasing dyspnoea, fatigue, oedema, weight gain)
- Double dose of diuretic or/and ACE inhibitor
- Temporarily reduce the dose of β blockers if increasing diuretic dose does not work
- Review patient in one to two weeks; if no improvement seek specialist advice
- In cases of serious deterioration halve the dose of β blocker
- Stop β blocker (rarely necessary; seek specialist advice)

Bradycardia
- Electrocardiogram to exclude heart block
- Consider pacemaker support if patient experiences severe bradycardia or atrioventricular block or sick sinus node soon after starting β blockers
- Review need, reduce or discontinue other heart rate slowing drugs—for example, digoxin, amiodarone, diltiazem
- Reduce dose of β blocker. Discontinuation is rarely necessary

Severe decompensated heart failure, pulmonary oedema, shock
- Admit patient to hospital
- Discontinue β blocker if inotropic support is needed or symptomatic hypotension/bradycardia is observed
- Inotropic support may be needed

Adapted from European Society of Cardiology guidelines (2005)

Study of effect of digoxin on mortality and morbidity in patients with heart failure*

Number of participants: 6800
Design: prospective, randomised, double blind, placebo controlled
Participants: left ventricular ejection fraction <45%
Intervention: randomised to digoxin (0.125–0.500 μg) or placebo; follow-up at 37 months
Results:
- Reduced admissions to hospital owing to heart failure (greater absolute and relative benefits in the patients with resistant symptoms and more severe impairment of left ventricular systolic function)
- No effect on overall survival

*Digitalis Investigation Group. *N Engl J Med* 1997;336:525–33)

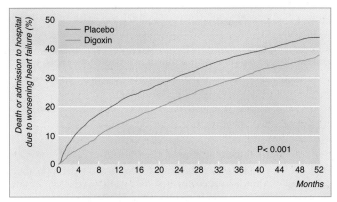

Incidence of death or admission to hospital due to worsening heart failure in two groups of patients: those receiving digoxin and those receiving placebo. Adapted from the Digitalis Investigation Group. *N Engl J Med* 1997;336:525–33

ABC of heart failure

The prospective randomized study of ibopamine on mortality and efficacy (PRIME II) trial examined ibopamine, a weak inotrope, in patients with chronic heart failure who were already receiving standard treatment. An excess mortality was shown, particularly in those with severe symptoms; this was possibly related to an excess of arrhythmias. A previous trial evaluating intermittent dobutamine infusions in patients with chronic heart failure was stopped prematurely because of excess mortality in the group taking dobutamine. Xamoterol, a β receptor antagonist with mild agonist inotropic effects, also failed to show any positive benefits in patients with heart failure. Other inotropic agents that have been used include milrinone and enoximone, but none has shown a survival benefit.

In overall terms, no evidence exists at present to support the use of oral catecholamine receptor (or postreceptor pathway) stimulants in the treatment of chronic heart failure. Digoxin remains the only (albeit weak) positive inotrope that is valuable in the management of chronic heart failure.

Antithrombotic treatment

In patients with chronic heart failure the incidence of stroke and thromboembolism is significantly higher in the presence of atrial and left ventricular dilatation, particularly in severe left ventricular dysfunction. Nevertheless, there is conflicting evidence of the benefit from routine treatment of patients with heart failure who are in sinus rhythm with antithrombotic treatment, though anticoagulation should be considered in the presence of mobile ventricular thrombus, atrial fibrillation, and severe cardiac impairment.

The small warfarin/aspirin study in heart failure (WASH) did not show the expected benefit of routine anticoagulation in sinus rhythm patients. Two large scale prospective randomised controlled trials of antithrombotic treatment in heart failure have been carried out; (preliminary) results of the WATCH study (a trial of warfarin and antiplatelet therapy) do not suggest any benefit of routine anticoagulation, though recruitment for the study was lower than anticipated. The results of the warfarin versus aspirin in reduced cardiac ejection fraction (WARCEF) study are awaited with interest. At present, therefore, the routine use of anticoagulation for patients with heart failure in sinus rhythm either owing to ischaemia or dilated cardiomyopathy cannot be advocated.

The combination of atrial fibrillation and heart failure (or evidence of left ventricular systolic dysfunction on echocardiography) is associated with a particularly high risk of thromboembolism, which is reduced by two thirds by long term treatment with warfarin. Formal anticoagulation is therefore strongly advocated in heart failure with atrial fibrillation, unless there are major contraindications. Similarly a definite history of thromboembolism is a powerful indication for anticoagulation.

Aspirin seems to have little effect on the risk of thromboembolism and overall mortality in such patients, but there is a suggestion of increased admissions to hospital for heart failure with aspirin compared with warfarin.

Antiarrhythmic treatment

Chronic heart failure and atrial fibrillation
Restoration and long term maintenance of sinus rhythm is less successful in the presence of severe structural heart disease, particularly when the atrial fibrillation is longstanding. In patients with a deterioration in symptoms that is associated with recent onset atrial fibrillation, treatment with amiodarone increases the long term success rate of cardioversion. β blockers

Meta-analysis of trials comparing warfarin with aspirin on death, myocardial infarction, and stroke in patients with heart failure and left ventricular systolic dysfunction. Adapted from Cleland J, et al. *Eur J Heart Failure* 2004;6:501–8

Meta-analysis of trials comparing warfarin with aspirin on admission to hospital for heart failure in patients with heart failure and left ventricular systolic dysfunction. Adapted from Cleland J, et al. *Eur J Heart Failure* 2004;6:501–8

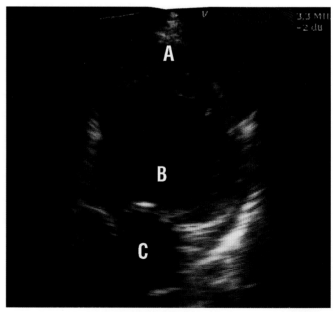

Echocardiogram showing thrombus at left ventricular apex in patient with dilated cardiomyopathy (A = thrombus, B = left ventricle, C = left atrium)

with or without digoxin are otherwise appropriate for controlling ventricular rate in most patients with heart failure and chronic atrial fibrillation, with the addition of amiodarone in resistant cases. Rate limiting calcium antagonists (verapamil and diltiazem) are best avoided because of their negative inotropic effects.

Chronic heart failure and ventricular arrhythmias

Ventricular arrhythmias are a common cause of death in severe heart failure. Precipitating or aggravating factors should therefore be dealt with, including electrolyte disturbance (for example, hypokalaemia, hypomagnesaemia), digoxin toxicity, drugs causing electrical instability (for example, antiarrhythmic drugs, antidepressants), and continued or recurrent myocardial ischaemia.

Amiodarone is effective for the symptomatic control of ventricular arrhythmias in chronic heart failure, though most studies have reported that long term antiarrhythmic treatment with amiodarone has a neutral effect on survival. An Argentinian trial (the GESICA study) of empirical amiodarone in patients with chronic heart failure, however, reported that active treatment was associated with a 28% reduction in total mortality, though this trial included a high incidence of patients with non-ischaemic heart failure. In contrast, in the survival trial of antiarrhythmic therapy in congestive heart failure (CHF-STAT), amiodarone did not improve overall survival, though there was a significant (46%) reduction in cardiac death and admission to hospital in the patients with non-ischaemic chronic heart failure. More recently, the sudden cardiac death in heart failure trial (SCD HeFT) showed no evidence of benefit from the routine use of amiodarone in heart failure patients without evidence of arrhythmias, in contrast with significant mortality benefit with implantable defibrillator therapy (see chapter 7). In general, amiodarone should probably be reserved for patients with chronic heart failure who also have symptomatic ventricular arrhythmias. Even in those with an implantable cardioverter defibrillator, amiodarone may be useful in reducing symptomatic arrhythmias and frequency of discharges from an implantable cardioverter defibrillator. The neutral results of the SCD HeFT amiodarone arm do at least suggest that it is safe to use amiodarone, even if it does not improve survival.

This chapter was adapted from the corresponding one in the first edition written by CR Gibbs, MK Davies, and GYH Lip. Our colleague's previous contribution is gratefully acknowledged.

The use of class I antiarrhythmic agents in patients with atrial fibrillation and chronic heart failure substantially increases the risk of mortality

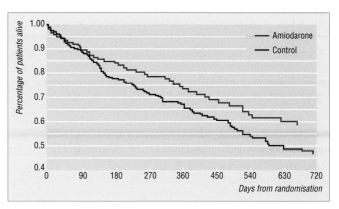

Survival curves from GESICA trial, showing difference between patients taking amiodarone and controls. Adapted from Doval HC, et al. *Lancet* 1994;344:493–8

Further reading

- Bardy GH, Lee KL, Poole JE, Packer DL, Boineau R, Domanski M, et al. Amiodarone or an implantable cardioverter-defibrillator for congestive heart failure. *N Engl J Med* 2005;352:225–37.
- Digitalis Investigation Group. The effect of digoxin on mortality and morbidity in patients with heart failure. *N Engl J Med* 1997;336:525–33.
- Lip GYH. Intracardiac thrombus formation in cardiac impairment: investigation and the role of anticoagulant therapy. *Postgrad Med J* 1996;72:731–8.
- Packer M, Bristow MR, Cohn JN, Colucci WS, Fowler MB, Gilbert EM, et al. Effect of carvedilol on morbidity and mortality in patients with chronic heart failure. *N Engl J Med* 1996;334:1349–55.
- Packer M, Fowler MB, Roecker EB, Coats AJ, Katus HA, Krum H, et al. Effect of carvedilol on the morbidity of patients with severe chronic heart failure: results of the carvedilol prospective randomized cumulative survival (COPERNICUS study). *Circulation* 2002;106:2194–9.
- Poole-Wilson PA, Swedberg K, Cleland JGF, Di Lenarda A, Hanrath P, Komajda M, et al. Comparison of carvedilol and metoprolol on clinical outcomes in patients with chronic heart failure in the carvedilol or metoprolol European trial (COMET): randomised controlled trial. *Lancet* 2003;362:7–13.

10 Acute and chronic management strategies

Acute and chronic management strategies in heart failure are aimed at improving both symptoms and prognosis, though management in individual patients will depend on the underlying aetiology and the severity of the condition. It is imperative that the diagnosis of heart failure is accompanied by an urgent attempt to establish its cause because timely intervention may greatly improve the prognosis in selected cases-for example, in patients with severe aortic stenosis.

Management of acute heart failure

Assessment
Common presenting features include anxiety, tachycardia, and dyspnoea. Pallor and hypotension are present in more severe cases: the triad of hypotension (systolic blood pressure <90 mm Hg), oliguria, and low cardiac output constitutes a diagnosis of cardiogenic shock. Severe acute heart failure and cardiogenic shock may be related to an extensive myocardial infarction, sustained cardiac arrhythmias (for example, atrial fibrillation or ventricular tachycardia), or mechanical problems (for example, acute papillary muscle rupture or postinfarction ventricular septal defect).

Severe acute heart failure is a medical emergency, and effective management requires an assessment of the underlying cause, improvement of the haemodynamic status, relief of pulmonary congestion, and improved tissue oxygenation. Clinical and radiographic assessment of these patients provides a guide to severity and prognosis: the Killip classification grades the severity of acute and chronic heart failure.

Treatment
Basic measures should include sitting the patient in an upright position with high concentration oxygen delivered via a face mask. Close observation and frequent reassessment are required in the early hours of treatment, and patients with acute severe heart failure, or refractory symptoms, should be monitored in a high dependency unit. Urinary catheterisation facilitates accurate assessment of fluid balance, while arterial blood gases provide valuable information about oxygenation and acid-base balance. The "base excess" is a guide to actual tissue perfusion in patients with acute heart failure: a worsening (more negative) base excess generally indicates lactic acidosis, which is related to anaerobic metabolism and is a poor prognostic feature. Correction of hypoperfusion will correct the metabolic acidosis; bicarbonate infusions should be reserved for only the most refractory cases.

Intravenous loop diuretics, such as furosemide (frusemide), induce transient venodilatation when administered to patients with pulmonary oedema, and this may lead to symptomatic improvement even before the onset of diuresis. Loop diuretics also increase the renal production of vasodilator prostaglandins. This additional benefit is antagonised by the administration of prostaglandin inhibitors, such as non-steroidal anti-inflammatory drugs, and these agents should be avoided where possible. Parenteral opiates or opioids (morphine or diamorphine) are an important adjunct in the management of severe acute heart failure by relieving anxiety, pain, and distress and reducing myocardial oxygen demand. Intravenous opiates and opioids also produce transient venodilatation, thus reducing preload, cardiac filling pressures, and pulmonary congestion.

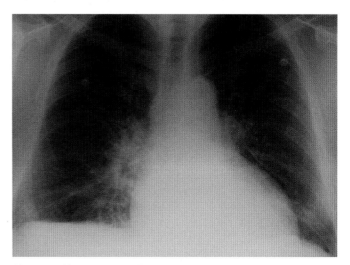

Chest x ray film in patient with acute pulmonary oedema

Killip classification

Class	Clinical features	Hospital mortality (%)
I	No signs of left ventricular dysfunction	6
II	S3 gallop with or without mild to moderate pulmonary congestion	30
III	Acute severe pulmonary oedema	40
IV	Shock syndrome	80–90

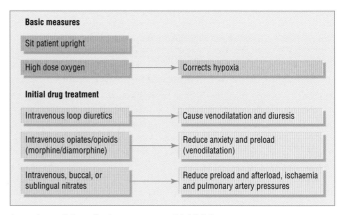

Acute heart failure: basic measures and initial drug treatment

Weighing the patient daily is valuable in monitoring the response to treatment

Nitrates (sublingual, buccal, and intravenous) may also reduce preload and cardiac filling pressures and are particularly valuable in patients with both angina and heart failure. Sodium nitroprusside is a potent, directly acting vasodilator, which is normally reserved for refractory cases of acute heart failure. Intravenous nitrate infusion should be considered for all patients with acute pulmonary oedema who do not respond rapidly to diuretics and opiates.

Short term inotropic support
In cases of severe refractory heart failure in which the cardiac output remains critically low, the circulation can be supported for a critical period of time with inotropic agents. For example, dobutamine and dopamine have positive inotropic actions, acting on the β_1 receptors in cardiac muscle. Phosphodiesterase inhibitors (for example, enoximone) are less commonly used, and long term use of these agents is associated with increased mortality. Intravenous aminophylline is now rarely used for treating acute heart failure. Inotropic agents in general increase the potential for cardiac arrhythmias.

Ventilation
In cases where pulmonary oedema fails to respond to medical treatment as outlined above, and the patient is becoming exhausted, ventilation should be considered. Non-invasive ventilation-continuous positive airways pressure (CPAP) or non-invasive positive pressure ventilation (NPPV) have been shown to reduce the need for airway intubation and invasive ventilation, though there is some concern that the risk of new myocardial infarction may be increased. Intubation and formal invasive ventilation is needed for resistant pulmonary oedema and when respiratory arrest occurs. It can be difficult to "wean" heart failure patients off ventilators once intubation has occurred, and an advance decision as to whether such treatment would be appropriate should be made in patients with known severe heart failure.

Newer agents-levosimendan and nesiritide
Levosimendan acts as a calcium sensitiser and has been shown to improve myocardial contractility without increasing oxygen demand. In the levosimendan infusion versus dobutamine in severe low output heart failure (LIDO) study, patients with severe low output cardiac failure were randomised to treatment with either intravenous levosimendan or dobutamine infusions; significantly more patients improved haemodynamically on the levosimendan, and 180 day mortality was also significantly lower (26% v 38%). Preliminary results from further studies unfortunately do not look so promising.

Nesiritide is a brain natriuretic peptide analogue that has been shown to lead to haemodynamic improvements in patients with acute severe heart failure. This has led it to its widespread use in North America; recent reports, however, suggest its use is associated with a 1.8-fold increase in mortality, so its use is likely to be curbed unless its safety can be proved.

Neither levosimendan nor nesiritide is licensed for use in the UK at present, and both drugs can worsen hypotension, which is a common problem in acute severe heart failure.

Chronic heart failure

Chronic heart failure can be "compensated" or "decompensated." In compensated heart failure, symptoms are stable, and many overt features of fluid retention and pulmonary oedema are absent. Decompensated heart failure refers to a deterioration, which may present either as an acute episode of pulmonary oedema or as lethargy and malaise, a

Intravenous inotropes and circulatory assist devices
- Short term support with intravenous inotropes or circulatory assist devices, or both, may temporarily improve haemodynamic status and peripheral perfusion
- Such support can act as a bridge to corrective valve surgery or cardiac transplantation in acute and chronic heart failure

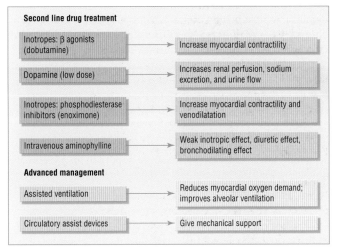

Second line drug treatment and advanced management in acute heart failure

Supervised exercise programmes are of proved benefit, and regular exercise should be encouraged in patients with chronic stable heart failure

reduction in exercise tolerance, and increasing breathlessness on exertion or increasing oedema/weight. The cause or causes of decompensation should be considered and identified; they may include recurrent ischaemia, arrhythmias, infections (especially chest), and electrolyte disturbance. Atrial fibrillation is common, and poor control of ventricular rate during exercise, despite adequate control at rest, should be dealt with.

Common features of chronic heart failure include breathlessness and reduced exercise tolerance, and management is directed at relieving these symptoms and improving quality of life. Secondary but important objectives are to improve prognosis and reduce hospital admissions.

Initial management

Non-pharmacological and lifestyle measures should be examined-particularly compliance. Loop diuretics are valuable if there is evidence of fluid overload, though these may be reduced once salt and water retention has been treated. Angiotensin converting enzyme (ACE) inhibitors should be introduced at an early stage, in the absence of clear contraindications.

Angiotensin II receptor antagonists are an appropriate alternative. β blockers (carvedilol, bisoprolol) are increasingly used in stable patients, though these drugs must be started at a low dose with cautious titration under specialist supervision. Oral digoxin has a role in patients with left ventricular systolic impairment, in sinus rhythm, who remain symptomatic despite optimal doses of diuretics and ACE inhibitors. Warfarin should be considered in patients with atrial fibrillation.

Education, counselling, and support

- A role is emerging for heart failure liaison nurses in educating and supporting patients and their families, promoting long term compliance, and supervising treatment changes in the community
- Depression is common, underdiagnosed, and often undertreated; counselling is therefore important for patients and families, and the newer antidepressants (particularly the selective serotonin reuptake inhibitors) seem to be well tolerated and are useful in selected patients

Severe congestive heart failure

Despite conventional treatment with diuretics and angiotensin converting enzyme inhibitors, hospital admission may be necessary for patients with severe congestive heart failure. Fluid restriction is important-fluid intake should be reduced to 1-1.5 litres/24 hours, and dietary salt restriction may be helpful.

Short term bed rest is valuable until signs and symptoms improve: rest reduces the metabolic demand and increases renal perfusion, thus improving diuresis. Though bed rest potentiates the action of diuretics, it increases the risk of venous thromboembolism, and prophylactic subcutaneous heparin or low molecular weight heparin should be considered in immobile inpatients.

Full anticoagulation is not advocated routinely unless concurrent atrial fibrillation is present. Intravenous loop diuretics may be administered to overcome the short term problem of gut oedema and reduced absorption of tablets.

In cases of severe fluid overload, furosemide given as an infusion rather than as boluses may have greater diuretic efficacy and cause less urinary urgency. The greater total diuresis over a 24 hour period can help reduce length of hospital stay. Low dose spironolactone (25 mg) improves morbidity and mortality in severe (New York Heart Association class IV) heart failure when it is combined with conventional treatment (loop diuretics and angiotensin converting enzyme

Management of chronic heart failure

General advice
- Counselling-about symptoms and compliance
- Social activity and employment
- Vaccination (influenza, pneumococcal)
- Contraception

General measures
- Diet (for example, reduce salt and fluid intake)
- Stop smoking
- Reduce alcohol intake
- Take exercise

Treatment options—pharmacological
- Diuretics (loop and thiazide)
- ACE inhibitors
- Angiotensin receptor antagonists
- β blockers
- Digoxin
- Aldosterone antagonists
- Vasodilators (hydralazine/nitrates)
- Anticoagulation
- Antiarrhythmic agents
- Positive inotropic agents

Treatment options-devices and surgery
- Revascularisation (percutaneous transluminal coronary angioplasty and coronary artery bypass graft)
- Valve replacement (or repair)
- Pacemaker or implantable cardiodefibrillator
- Ventricular assist devices
- Heart transplantation

Treatment of left ventricular systolic dysfunction
- Confirm diagnosis by echocardiography
- If possible, discontinue aggravating drugs (for example non-steroidal anti-inflammatory drugs)
- Address non-pharmacological and lifestyle measures

Symptomatic → Add loop diuretic (for example furosemide) → Angiotensin converting enzyme inhibitor → Consider β blocker* in patients with chronic, stable condition →

Asymptomatic → Angiotensin converting enzyme inhibitor

Persisting clinical features of heart failure
Options
- Optimise dose of loop diuretic
- Low dose spironolactone (25 mg once a day)
- Digoxin
- Combine loop and thiazide diuretics
- Oral nitrates/hydralazine

Atrial fibrillation
Options
- Digoxin
- β blocker (if not already given)
- Warfarin

Angina
Options
- β blocker (if not already given)
- Oral nitrates
- Calcium antagonist (for example amlodipine)

Consider specialist referral in patients with atrial fibrillation (electrical cardioversion or other antiarrhythmic agents - for example amiodarone - may be indicated), angina (coronary angiography and revascularisation may be indicated), or persistent or severe symptoms

In the United Kindom carvedilol, bisoprolol, and nebivolol are now licensed to treat heart failure

*Initial low dose (for example carvedilol, bisoprolol, metoprolol) with cautious titration under expert supervision.

Example of management algorithm for left ventricular dysfunction

inhibitors) and can also aid in diuresis. Potassium concentrations should be closely monitored after the addition of spironolactone. In cases where oedema is still resistant to the above treatments, a thiazide or thiazide-like diuretic (bendroflumethiazide or metolazone) may be added also, though close monitoring is needed due to the risk of rising urea and creatinine concentrations and hypokalaemia and hyponatraemia.

In resistant cases, haemofiltration may play a part in mobilising massive peripheral oedema, though availability of this is limited at present.

Special procedures

Intra-aortic balloon pumping and mechanical devices
Intra-aortic balloon counterpulsation and left ventricular assist devices are used as bridges to corrective valve surgery, cardiac transplantation, or coronary artery bypass surgery in the presence of poor cardiac function. Mechanical devices are indicated if there is a possibility of spontaneous recovery (for example, peripartum cardiomyopathy, myocarditis) or as a bridge to cardiac surgery (for example, ruptured mitral papillary muscle, postinfarction ventricular septal defect) or transplantation. Intra-aortic balloon counterpulsation is the most commonly used form of mechanical support.

Revascularisation and other operative strategies
Impaired ventricular function in itself is not an absolute contraindication to cardiac surgery, though the operative risks are increased. Ischaemic heart disease is the most common precursor of chronic heart failure in Britain; coronary ischaemia should be identified and revascularisation considered with coronary artery bypass surgery or occasionally percutaneous coronary angioplasty. The concept of "hibernating" myocardium is increasingly recognised, though the most optimal and practical methods of identifying hibernation remain open to debate. Magnetic resonance imaging scans with gadolinium, nuclear medicine techniques, especially positron emission tomography (PET scanning), and stress echo have all been used to identify hibernating myocardium. Revascularisation of hibernating myocardium may lead to an improvement in the overall left ventricular function and may also help concomitant symptoms of angina.

Correction of valve disease, most commonly in severe aortic stenosis or mitral incompetence (not secondary to left ventricular dilatation), relieves a mechanical cause of heart failure; closure of an acute ventricular septal defect or mitral valve surgery for acute mitral regurgitation, complicating a myocardial infarction, may be lifesaving. Surgical excision of a left ventricular aneurysm (aneurysectomy) is appropriate in selected cases. Novel surgical procedures such as extensive ventricular reduction (Batista operation) and cardiomyoplasty have been associated with successful outcome in a small number of patients, though the high mortality and the limited evidence of substantial benefit has restricted the widespread use of these procedures.

Cardiac transplantation
The outcome in cardiac transplantation is now good, with long term improvements in survival and quality of life in patients with severe heart failure. Though the demand for cardiac transplantation has increased over recent years, the number of transplant operations has remained stable, owing primarily to limited availability of donor organs.

The procedure now carries a perioperative mortality of less than 10%, with approximate one, five, and 10 year survival rates

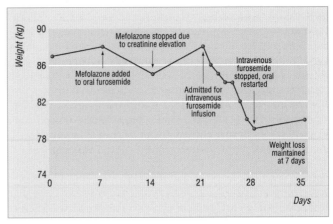

Chart showing weight loss after intravenous infusion of furosemide

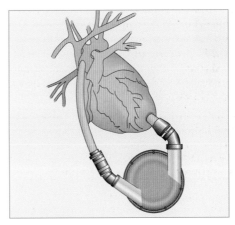

Left ventricular assist device

Transplantation in adults

Indications
- End stage heart failure for example, ischaemic heart disease and dilated cardiomyopathy
- Rarely, restrictive cardiomyopathy and peripartum cardiomyopathy
- Congenital heart disease (often combined heart-lung transplantation is required)
- End stage valve disease with severe left ventricular dilatation and dysfunction

Absolute contraindications
- Recent malignancy (other than basal cell and squamous cell carcinoma of the skin)
- Active infection (including HIV, hepatitis B, hepatitis C with liver disease)
- Systemic disease that is likely to affect life expectancy
- Severe pulmonary vascular resistance

Relative contraindications
- Recent pulmonary embolism
- Symptomatic peripheral vascular disease
- Obesity
- Renal impairment
- Psychosocial problems for example, lack of social support, poor compliance, psychiatric illness
- Age >60-65

of 92%, 75%, and 60% respectively (much better outcomes than with optimal drug treatment, which is associated with a one year mortality of 30-50% in advanced heart failure). Cardiac transplantation should be considered in patients with an estimated one year survival of <50%. Well selected patients aged >55-60 have survival rates comparable with those of younger patients. Patients need strong social and psychological support; transplant liaison nurses are valuable in this role.

The long term survival of the transplanted human heart is compromised by accelerated graft atherosclerosis, which results in small vessel coronary artery disease and an associated deterioration in left ventricular performance. This can occur as early as three months and is the major cause of graft loss after the first year. The anti-rejection regimens currently used may result in an acceleration of pre-existing atherosclerotic vascular disease-hence the exclusion of patients who already have severe peripheral vascular disease. Rejection is now a less serious problem, with the use of ciclosporin and other immunosuppressants. Nevertheless, the supply of donors limits the procedure and the number of heart transplants performed in the UK is declining. The UK transplant database (2000-3) indicates that 13% of patients listed for transplantation die on the waiting list, with 69% receiving transplants at two years (65% within 12 months). Though ventricular assist devices may be valuable during the wait for transplantation, the routine use of xenotransplants is unlikely in the short or medium term.

This chapter was adapted from the corresponding one in the first edition written by T Millane, G Jackson, CR Gibbs, and GYH Lip. Our colleagues' previous contribution is gratefully acknowledged.

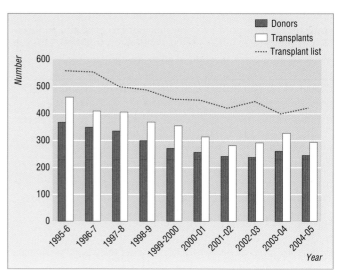

Number of donors, transplants and patients on the active cardiothoracic transplant list in the UK. Adapted from UK Transplant data

Further reading

- American College of Cardiology/American Heart Association Task Force Report Guidelines for the evaluation and management of heart failure. *J Am Coll Cardiol* 1995;26:1376-98.
- Dormans TPJ, van Meyel JJM, Gerlag PGG, Tan Y, Russel FGM, Smits P. Diuretic efficacy of high dose furosemide in severe heart failure: bolus versus continuous infusion. *J Am Coll Cardiol* 1996;28:376-82.
- Follath F, Cleland JG, Just H, Papp JG, Scholz H, Peuhkurinen K, et al. Efficacy and safety of intravenous levosimendan compared with dobutamine in severe low-output heart failure (the LIDO study): a randomised double-blind trial. *Lancet* 2002;360:196-202.
- Hunt SA. Current status of cardiac transplantation. *JAMA* 1998:280:1692-8.
- Remme WJ. The treatment of heart failure. The Task Force of the Working Group on Heart Failure of the European Society of Cardiology. *Eur Heart J* 1997;18:736-53.
- Topol EJ. Nesiritide-not verified. *N Engl J Med* 2005;353:113-6.

11 Specialist heart failure nursing services

Specialist heart failure nurses are a key component of heart failure services and represent a crucial component of any multidisciplinary heart failure management programmes. Often such interventions complement clinic based care for patients with heart failure. Specialist nurses fulfil many roles in the management of these patients.

In one recent study, a clinic plus home based intervention was superior to "usual care" in reducing unplanned readmission for any cause (22% v 44%). It was associated with a 45% reduction in the risk of death or readmission after adjustment for potential confounders, fewer days of recurrent hospital stay (108 v 459 days), a greater uptake of β blocker therapy (56% v 18%), and improved adherence to sodium restrictions during six month's follow-up.

Education and emotional support

Even when a physician takes time to explain the diagnosis of heart failure and the options for treatment in some detail, recall of such information in this group of predominantly elderly patients is often poor, and reinforcement of the messages along with clarification and discussion may be best done by a nurse. Patients can often feel intimidated by even the most sensitive doctors and will often express their fears and concerns more openly to nurses.

Poor adherence to prescribed treatment is a common reason for decompensation of heart failure and hospital admissions, and this is an obvious target for education programmes. Reasons for not taking drugs can be explored, and genuine problems can be discussed with physicians, with possible changes in dose or type of drugs ensuing.

Education of relatives and carers of patients, with discussion of realistic expectations, can also be neglected in traditional models of care, and specialist nurses can be useful in filling this gap. Emotional support for both patients and carers may help to motivate patients to comply with treatment and to cope with their disease and its impact on their lives. As well as being someone to turn to, the nurse may also be able to give more practical support with arrangement of drugs, meals, and transport and help with applications for benefit claims.

Despite the advances in treatment, mortality in patients with heart failure is still high, and emotional and practical support for the newly bereaved has often been poor. Help with funeral arrangements and in the first few days can be invaluable, especially for those who may be otherwise socially isolated.

Optimisation of medication and monitoring for side effects

With angiotensin converting enzyme (ACE) inhibitors (or angiotensin receptor antagonists) and β blockers now established incontrovertibly as standard treatment for those with all grades of heart failure due to left ventricular systolic dysfunction, and many patients also requiring spironolactone in addition to other medications—for example, aspirin, statins, diuretics, antihypertensives—polypharmacy is now the norm. ACE inhibitors

---

The roles of specialist heart failure nurses
- Education and emotional support
- Optimisation of medication and monitoring for side effects
- Early detection of deterioration and prevention of hospital admission
- Terminal care

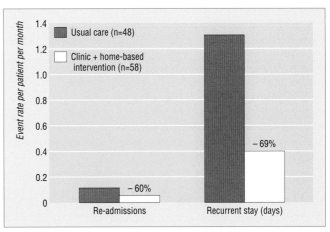

Comparison of recurrent hospital admission and associated stay. Adapted form Thompson DR, et al *Eur J Heart Fail* 2005;7:377–84

Education is important
- Surveys of the general public have suggested that many think that a diagnosis of heart failure equates to one of cardiac arrest and leads to imminent death
- In view of this, simply telling a patient that he or she has heart failure without further explanation is likely to cause confusion and distress

and (especially) β blockers require multiple dose titration steps, which may take several months even with the same frequency of titration steps as used in clinical trials.

In the traditional system found in the NHS, the process may take even longer because cardiology outpatient appointments in hospitals are often not available at intervals of less than three months, and general practitioners have been reluctant to titrate and monitor patients in the community, partly because the use of β blockers is contrary to the training they received in medical school. In this context, the use of spironolactone is also potentially dangerous because blood testing for renal function and hyperkalaemia is labour intensive and may not be done as assiduously as in the trials. For these reasons, there is evidence that many patients never receive full evidence based doses of medication, if the appropriate treatments are initiated at all.

In nurse led clinics, in either a hospital or community setting, or even in patients' own homes, medication can be titrated using guidelines based on clinical trial protocols, with monitoring done as vigilantly as it is in clinical trials. Thus, patients will be much more likely to receive full dose and appropriate treatment.

In the traditional models of care for patients with heart failure, many patients stopped taking drugs because of concerns about side effects and not knowing what medications were for. Communications between primary and secondary care were often suboptimal, leading to medications that had been stopped because of adverse effects being inadvertently re-started. The heart failure specialist nurse is well positioned to be able to check what medications are actually being taken by patients, by checking medication bottles and packets and counting the numbers of tablets used between the date of issue and the present. Reasons for discrepancies can be explored and discussed. This may be best done in the patient's home, where the reasons may be clear—for example, a poorly mobile patient being prescribed large doses of diuretics when the toilet is upstairs. In this instance, urine bottles or a commode downstairs may greatly improve adherence to prescribed drugs.

In addition to achieving treatment targets, the nurse led clinics can also be used as a forum to continue the process of education about the condition and emphasise the use of non-pharmacological treatments such as weight management, salt and fluid intake, and exercise.

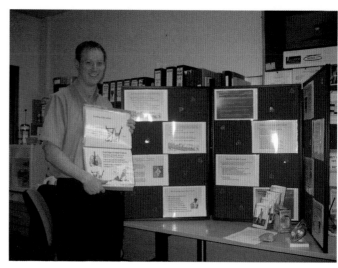
Heart failure specialist nurse during an information session

> **Specialist nurses in heart failure are well placed to assist in the titration of medication and monitoring for side effects and complications of treatment**

Early detection of deterioration and prevention of hospital admission

The large studies of nursing services in heart failure have concentrated on patients who have already had one admission for their disease. This is not surprising given that previous admission is the strongest predictor of future admission. There is also evidence that up to two thirds of readmissions with heart failure are due to "avoidable" factors such as inadequate prescription of appropriate therapy, poor adherence with treatment, poor recognition of clinical deterioration or poor response to it, poor social support, problems with caregivers and the home environment, and poor responsiveness of the traditional models of care. Urgent consultant review is rarely available, and even review by a general practitioner may be hard to arrange, especially for housebound patients. Also, medications may not be optimised or monitored as fully as desirable.

The many published trials of specialist nurse intervention in heart failure have all had slightly different entry criteria and interventions have varied. A common theme of the more successful trials, however, has been the provision of increased monitoring and improved education and individualised follow-up. Results from different countries and healthcare systems also seem

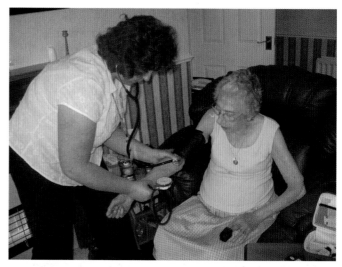
Heart failure specialist nurse monitoring a patient with severe heart failure at home. Note her ascites and muscular wasting. This type of patient finds travelling to a hospital clinic very difficult

to be comparable. One study involved a pharmacist intervention rather than nursing intervention, with telephone follow-up rather than home visits, and again reported positive results. Published studies consistently show a reduction in hospital readmissions and improvements in quality of life measures.

A study of intensive home based intervention in Glasgow found fewer readmissions for any reason (86 v 114), fewer admissions for heart failure (19 v 45), and fewer days in hospital (3.4 v 7.5 days). All the patients had been recruited into the study while they were in hospital for heart failure.

While frequent home visiting by a dedicated nurse might be the ideal option for patients, this is clearly extremely labour intensive and costly. Telephone contact is one option to reduce the number of visits needed; another is telemonitoring, with various clinical variables, such as weight, being measured either by the patient and entered on a computer, or in an automated manner, and further action taken if results are worrying. A recent study of home telemonitoring versus nurse telephone support or "usual care" showed significantly lower mortality in both telemonitoring and telephone support groups, mortality being reduced by 29% and 27%. Though rates of admission to hospital were similar in the telemonitoring and telephone support groups, stays were shorter in the telemonitoring group, perhaps because deterioration was picked up earlier and was easier to treat in hospital.

The use of telephone support, home visiting, and telemonitoring may vary considerably according to geographical factors (visiting being more difficult in isolated areas) and local availability of resources. Home telemonitoring is also likely to evolve over the coming years, perhaps including fingerprick blood testing—for example, for natriuretic peptides.

Terminal care

Despite therapeutic advances, the morbidity and mortality of heart failure remain high. Though the mode of death in about half of patients is sudden (due to arrhythmia or a new ischaemic event), in the other half it is due to progressive heart failure. Most such patients die in hospital and often have a distressing final illness course, including out of hours visits from doctors who may be unaware of the patients' previous disease course, repeated ambulance journeys to hospital, long waits on trolleys in the emergency departments, and suboptimal care delivered within the hospital by non-specialists. This is often against the wishes of patients, who, when questioned, often say they would prefer to die at home rather than in hospital.

The role of the hospice

In contrast, care for patients with malignancy in the terminal phase has been of considerably higher quality in recent years, with specialist nurses often able to deliver palliative care within the home. The hospice movement has been popular with patients and their families and is widely accepted as the best model. However, at least in the UK, hospices have generally been funded by charitable bodies, often with a specific remit to care for patients with malignancy, and hospice facilities have been denied to those with heart failure (and also end stage respiratory and neurological disease). This is despite the prognosis of heart failure from first admission being worse than that for many common cancers. As well as the funding issues, there is also the problem of capacity, in that palliative care services in many areas are already working to full capacity with patients with malignancy.

Those who have worked in palliative care services with patients with heart failure and those with cancer have often been surprised at the often more unpredictable disease course in heart failure, with patients often experiencing several

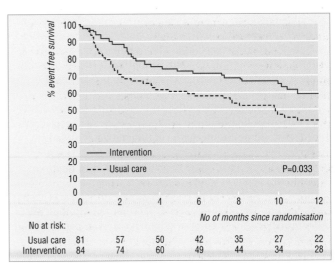

Time to first event (death from any cause or hospital admission for heart failure) in usual care and nurse intervention groups in the Glasgow study. From Blue L, et al. *BMJ*;323:715–8

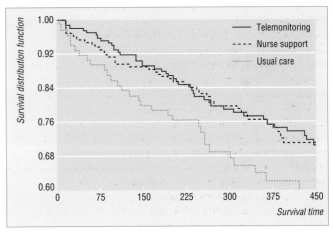

In the trans-European network home care management system study, the absolute difference in mortality at one year was 16% to 18%. Adapted from Cleland JG, et al. *J Am Coll Cardiol* 2005;45:1654–64

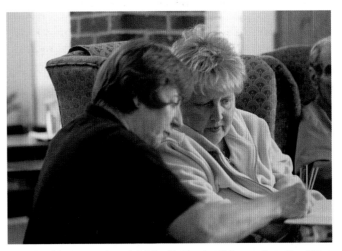

Staff nurse with a patient at St Michael's Hospice, St Leonards-on-Sea, UK. With permission from John Cole/Science Photo Library

"crises"—for example, due to arrhythmias or infections—with reasonable recovery of functional status afterwards. This is in contrast with the often more steady decline of patients with malignancy. It is also hard to predict length of survival of patients with heart failure; some patients with even extremely severe disease and symptoms continuing to live for many months, albeit with poor quality of life.

There is, therefore, great potential for the use of palliative care services in heart failure. In organising local services, it is logical to build on the strengths of local facilities already available. For example, if there is a well established cancer hospice facility, with funding available and staff willing to expand their remit, it would be logical for them to be involved. In other places, heart failure nurses may be the more obvious candidates to extend their service. To some extent, they will often have been involved in offering elements of palliative care from their first contact with their patients.

Patients with heart failure entering the terminal phase will often have associated symptoms of their underlying disease, such as angina, or associated disease, such as stroke, lower limb ischaemia, or leg ulceration. Pain management with opiates will be important, and opiates may also be of use in those with sleep difficulties. Those who develop resistance to the effects of oral diuretics may benefit from intravenous diuretics in the home or a hospice. Skin care is also an important issue in the terminal phase, especially in those with chronically oedematous legs and cachexia. All pressure areas need care, including elbows and even the neck and scalp in those unable to move. Air mattresses, frequent turning, and appropriate wound dressing may be delivered in the home or hospice. In the final phase, the presence of a healthcare worker around the clock to tend for patients' needs and distress may be invaluable.

Nutrition is often neglected in the final phase of illness and may contribute to the terminal decline. Patients with poor intestinal perfusion often have poor appetites, and it is important that what food they are able to eat is of good nutritional value. Appropriate advice at this stage may supersede advice previously given. For example, many with ischaemic heart disease will have been advised to use skimmed milk, but in the terminal phase of heart failure the calories of whole milk may be beneficial. For those who may have difficulty preparing food, advice on appropriate snacks and drinks may be particularly helpful. Institution of appropriate measures at an early stage, including "build up" drinks if needed, may help to prevent the development of pressure sores mentioned above.

Hospices may be able to provide both respite care for patients (and their relatives) and also care of the dying. Many patients, however, may want to die at home, and the option of both a hospice with inpatient facilities and a "hospice at home" service would be ideal. Additional day facilities can provide help with personal hygiene for those who have difficulty bathing at home and emotional support for patients and some period of rest for carers and relatives, who are often elderly and infirm.

Cost effectiveness of nursing services

Several studies have suggested that a specialist nurse led service could result in a 50% reduction of hospital bed use. Stewart and colleagues calculated that the cost of such a service is about equivalent to the saving made by a 40% reduction in bed use. Therefore a service that delivers a 50% or greater reduction will save the health service money—estimated at £169 000 per 1000 patients treated.

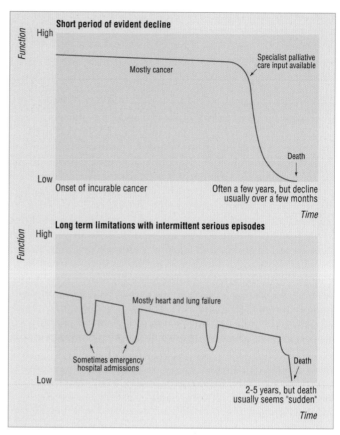

Disease trajectories of terminal conditions. Heart failure tends to follow the unpredictable course shown in the lower graph. Adapted from Murray SA, et al. *BMJ* 2005;330:1007–11

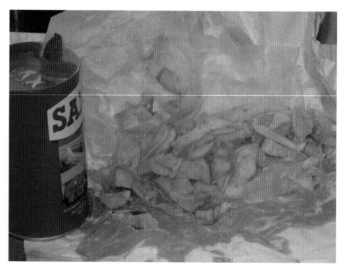

Patients often have small appetites but it is important that what they do eat is of nutritional value

Financial benefits

- Costs of admission to hospital account for about two thirds of health service expenditure on heart failure
- Multiple studies have shown that the readmission rates for patients with heart failure can be substantially reduced by a dedicated nursing service
- There is the potential for such services to yield considerable cost savings, in addition to the enormous benefits for the individual patients

Clinical effectiveness of nursing services

Meta-analysis of the effects of disease management programmes on hospital admission rates and mortality have been somewhat limited by the variable interventions used by trial investigators. Nurses have played a key role in all studies, with variable input from physicians, pharmacists, and social workers. A recent meta-analysis showed that strategies incorporating follow-up by a specialised multidisciplinary team reduced mortality (risk ratio 0.75, 95% confidence interval 0.59 to 0.96), heart failure hospitalisations (0.74, 0.63 to 0.87) and all-cause hospitalisations (0.81, 0.71 to 0.92). Those patients with nurse support who are admitted often have shorter hospital stays.

Training of nurses

The ideal candidate for a job as a specialist heart failure nurse would have experience of managing patients with heart failure and other cardiac conditions in hospital, nursing in a community setting, and ideally palliative care. Clearly there are few candidates (if any) with all these attributes, and therefore recruitment of more senior specialist nurses is likely to come from either hospital cardiology or the community. Training programmes need to consider this diversity of recruits' backgrounds to ensure they all feel confident in working in challenging new jobs.

Dedicated training programmes for more junior nurses to specialise in heart failure from an early stage in their careers would be highly beneficial and should be considered. The benefits a dedicated service can offer could then be made available to all patients, not just a selected few.

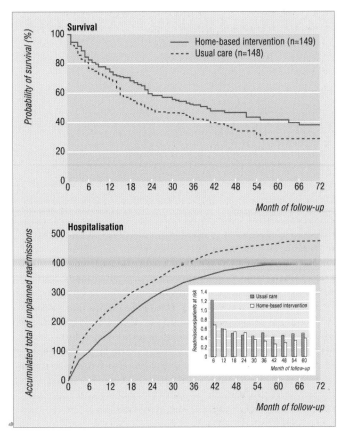

Effects of home based intervention on survival and hospitalisation of heart failure patients with at least one previous hospital admission. Adapted from Stewart S, Horowitz JD. *Circulation* 2002;105:2861–6

Further readng

- Cleland JG, Louis AA, Rigby AS, Janssens U, Balk AH; TEN-HMS Investigators. Noninvasive home telemonitoring for patients with heart failure at high risk of recurrent admission and death: the Trans-European Network-Home-Care Management System (TEN-HMS) study. *J Am Coll Cardiol* 2005;45:1654–64.
- Cleland JG, Cohen-Solal A, Aguilar JC, Dietz R, Eastaugh J, Follath F, Freemantle N, Gavazzi A, van Gilst WH, Hobbs FD, Korewicki J, Madeira HC, Preda I, Swedberg K, Widimsky J; IMPROVEMENT of Heart Failure Programme Committees and Investigators. Improvement programme in evaluation and management; Study Group on Diagnosis of the Working Group on Heart Failure of The European Society of Cardiology. Management of heart failure in primary care (the IMPROVEMENT of Heart Failure Programme): an international survey. *Lancet* 2002;360:1631–9.

- Murray SA, Kendall M, Boyd K, Sheikh A. Illness trajectories and palliative care. *BMJ* 2005;330:1007–11.
- Rich MW, Beckham V, Wittenberg C, Leven CL, Freedland KE, Carney RM. A multidisciplinary intervention to prevent the readmission of elderly patients with congestive heart failure. *N Engl J Med* 1995;333:1190–95.
- Stewart S, Blue L, Walker A, Morrison C, McMurray JJ. An economic analysis of specialist heart failure management in the UK—can we afford not to implement it? *Eur Heart J* 2002;23:1369–78.
- Blue L, Lang E, McMurray JJ, Davie AP, McDonagh TA, Murdoch DR, Petrie MC, Connolly E, Norrie J, Round CE, Ford I, Morrison CE. Randomised controlled trial of specialist nurse intervention in heart failure. *BMJ* 2001;323:715–8.
- McAlister FA, Stewart S, Ferrua S, McMurray JJV. Multidisciplinary strategies for the management of heart failure patients at high risk for admission. *J Am Coll Cardiol* 2004;44:819–19.

12 Heart failure with preserved systolic function

In elderly patients, the percentage admitted to hospital with heart failure-like symptoms and preserved systolic function may be as high as 35-45%.

The recent European Society of Cardiology guidelines provide definitions on "heart failure with preserved systolic function" (so called "diastolic heart failure"). A diagnosis of primary diastolic heart failure requires three conditions to be simultaneously satisfied:

- Presence of signs or symptoms of congestive heart failure
- Presence of normal or only mildly abnormal left ventricular systolic function (left ventricular ejection fraction 45–50%)
- Evidence of abnormal left ventricular relaxation, diastolic distensibility, or diastolic stiffness.

Furthermore, it is essential to exclude pulmonary disease.

It is important to emphasise that to make a diagnosis of heart failure with preserved systolic function, other differential diagnoses should be considered. Precipitating factors should be identified and corrected, in particular blood pressure should be controlled, tachyarrhythmias should be prevented and sinus rhythm restored whenever possible (for patients with atrial fibrillation). In other patients with atrial fibrillation, rate control is important.

Heart failure with preserved systolic function and heart failure due to diastolic dysfunction are not necessarily synonymous. The former diagnosis implies the evidence of preserved left ventricular ejection fraction and not that left ventricular diastolic dysfunction has been demonstrated.

The diagnosis of isolated diastolic heart failure requires evidence of abnormal diastolic function, which can be difficult to assess in the absence of any ideal echocardiographic parameter.

Echocardiographic features

At an early stage of diastolic dysfunction, there is typically a pattern of "impaired myocardial relaxation" with a decrease in peak transmitral E velocity, a compensatory increase in the atrial-induced (A) velocity, and, therefore, a decrease in the E:A ratio.

In patients with more advanced cardiac disease, there may be a pattern of "restrictive filling," with a raised peak E-velocity, a short E-deceleration time, and a markedly increased E:A ratio. The raised peak E velocity is due to raised left atrial pressure that causes an increase in the early diastolic transmitral pressure gradient.

In patients with an intermediate pattern between impaired relaxation and restrictive filling the E:A ratio and the deceleration time may be normal, a so called "pseudonormalised filling pattern." This pattern may be distinguished from normal filling by the demonstration of reduced peak E velocity by tissue Doppler imaging.

Thus the three filling patterns-impaired relaxation, pseudonormalised filling, and restrictive filling - represent mild, moderate, and severe diastolic dysfunction, respectively.

> We still lack prospective outcome studies that investigate if assessment of diastolic function by echocardiographic criteria may improve management of heart failure patients

> There is still uncertainty about the prevalence of diastolic dysfunction in patients with symptoms of heart failure and normal systolic function in the community

Assessment of left ventricular diastolic function

- To detect abnormalities of diastolic function in patients who present with congestive heart failure and normal left ventricular ejection fraction, and those with known systolic dysfunction
- To provide a non-invasive estimate of left ventricular diastolic pressure
- To diagnose constrictive pericarditis and restrictive cardiomyopathy

Differential diagnosis in a patient with heart failure and normal left ventricular ejection fraction

- Incorrect diagnosis of heart failure
- Inaccurate measurement of left ventricular ejection fraction
- Primary valvular disease
- Restrictive (infiltrative) cardiomyopathies
- Amyloidosis, sarcoidosis, haemochromatosis
- Pericardial constriction
- Episodic or reversible left ventricular systolic dysfunction
- Severe hypertension, myocardial ischaemia
- Heart failure associated with high metabolic demand (high output states)
- Anaemia, thyrotoxicosis, arteriovenous fistulas
- Chronic pulmonary disease with right heart failure
- Pulmonary hypertension associated with pulmonary vascular disorders
- Atrial myxoma
- Diastolic dysfunction of uncertain origin
- Obesity

Adapted from American College of Cardiology/American Heart Association 2005 guideline update for the diagnosis and management of chronic heart failure in the adult

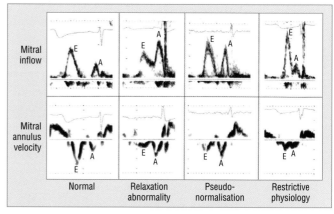

Mitral valve pulsed wave and tissue Doppler features in diastolic dysfunction. Adapted from Sohn DW, et al. *J Am Coll Cardiol* 1997;31:474–80

Management

The one large randomised clinical trial of patients with heart failure with preserved left ventricular ejection fraction is the candesartan in heart failure: assessment of reduction in mortality and morbidity-preserved (CHARM-preserved) trial. Patients with New York Heart Association functional class II-IV congestive heart failure and left verntricular ejection fraction >40% were randomised to candesartan (n=1514, target dose 32 mg once daily) or matching placebo (n=1509). In the trial, 22% of patients in the candesartan and 24% in the placebo group experienced cardiovascular death or hospital admission. Cardiovascular death did not differ between groups, but fewer patients in the candesartan group than in the placebo group were admitted to hospital for congestive heart failure. The conclusion was that candesartan had only a moderate impact in preventing these admissions among such patients.

Other ongoing clinical trials in such patients, such as the irbesartan in heart failure with preserved systolic function (I-PRESERVE) trial and the perindopril in elderly people with chronic heart failure (PEP-CHF) study, would inform our clinical management.

The European Society of Cardiology guidelines state that "there is no clear evidence that patients with primary diastolic heart failure benefit from any specific drug regimen." An important point is that those with correctable risk factors, such as poorly controlled hypertension, should have their blood pressure controlled, especially if there is left ventricular hypertrophy present. Similarly, associated arrhythmias, such as atrial fibrillation, require adequate rate control and other management-such as anticoagulation-as necessary.

Drug management

- Angiotensin converting enzyme (ACE) inhibitors may improve relaxation and cardiac distensibility directly and may have long term effects through their anti-hypertensive effects and regression of hypertrophy and fibrosis
- Diuretics may be necessary when episodes with fluid overload are present, but should be used cautiously so as not to lower preload excessively and thereby reduce stroke volume and cardiac output
- β blockade could be instituted to lower heart rate and increase the diastolic filling period
- Verapamil-type calcium antagonists may be used for the same reason. Some studies with verapamil have shown a functional improvement in patients with hypertrophic cardiomyopathy
- A high dose of an angiotensin receptor blocker may reduce admissions to hospital.

Other European Society of Cardiology recommendations for the management of such patients are summarised in the adjacent box.

There is still little evidence on how best to treat heart failure with preserved systolic function

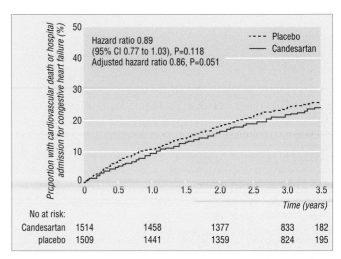

Survival curves from the CHARM-preserved study showing time to cardiovascular death or hospital admission for chronic heart failure. Adapted from Yusuf S, et al. *Lancet* 2003;362:777–81

European Society of Cardiology recommendations for treatment of patients with heart failure and normal left ventricular ejection fraction

- Control systolic and diastolic hypertension, in accordance with published guidelines
- Control ventricular rate in patients with atrial fibrillation
- Use diuretics to control pulmonary congestion and peripheral oedema
- Coronary revascularisation is reasonable in patients with coronary artery disease in whom symptomatic or demonstrable myocardial ischaemia is judged to be having an adverse effect on cardiac function
- Restoration and maintenance of sinus rhythm in patients with atrial fibrillation might be useful to improve symptoms
- The use of β adrenergic blocking agents, ACE inhibitors, angiotensin II receptor blockers, or calcium antagonists in patients with controlled hypertension might be effective to minimise symptoms of heart failure
- The use of digitalis to minimise symptoms of heart failure is not well established

Further reading

- European Study Group on Diastolic Heart Failure. How to diagnose diastolic heart failure. *European Heart Journal* 1998;19:990-1003.
- Yusuf S, Pfeffer MA, Swedberg K, Granger CB, Held P, McMurray JJ, et al. CHARM Investigators and Committees. Effects of candesartan in patients with chronic heart failure and preserved left-ventricular ejection fraction: the CHARM-preserved trial. *Lancet* 2003;362:777-81.

13 Heart failure in general practice

Management of heart failure in general practice has been hampered by difficulties in diagnosing the condition and by perceived difficulties in starting and monitoring treatment in the community. Nevertheless, improved access to diagnostic testing and increased confidence in the safety of treatment should help to improve the primary care management of heart failure. With improved survival and reduced admission rates (achieved by effective treatment) and a reduction in numbers of hospital beds, the community management of heart failure is likely to become increasingly important and the role of general practitioners, ideally working closely with specialist nursing teams, will become even more crucial.

Diagnostic accuracy

Heart failure is a difficult condition to diagnose clinically, and hence many patients thought by their general practitioners to have heart failure may not have any demonstrable abnormality of cardiac function on objective testing.

A study from Finland reported that only 32% of patients suspected of having heart failure by primary care doctors had definite heart failure (as determined by a clinical and radiographic scoring system). A recent study in the UK showed that only 35 of 122 patients referred to a "rapid access" clinic with a new diagnosis of heart failure fully met the definition of heart failure approved by the European Society of Cardiology— that is, appropriate symptoms, objective evidence of cardiac dysfunction, and response to treatment if doubt remained.

Similar findings have been reported in the echocardiographic heart of England screening (ECHOES) study, in which only about 22% of the patients with a diagnosis of heart failure in their general practice records had definite impairment of left ventricular systolic function on echocardiography, with a further 16% having borderline impairment. In addition, 23% had atrial fibrillation, with over half of these patients having normal left ventricular systolic contraction. Finally, patients may have clinical heart failure with normal systolic contraction and abnormal diastolic function; management of such patients with diastolic dysfunction is different to management of those with impaired systolic function.

Open access echocardiography and diagnosis

Because of the non-invasive nature of echocardiography, its high acceptability to patients, and its usefulness in assessing ventricular size and function, as well as valvar heart disease, many general practitioners now want direct access to echocardiography services for their patients. Though open access echocardiography services are available in some districts in the UK, many specialists still have reservations about introducing such services because of financial and staffing issues and concern that general practitioners would have difficulty interpreting technical reports. The cost of echocardiography (£50 to £100 per patient) is relatively small, however, compared with the cost of expensive treatment for heart failure that may not be needed. The cost is also small compared with the costs of hospital admission, which may be avoided by appropriate early treatment.

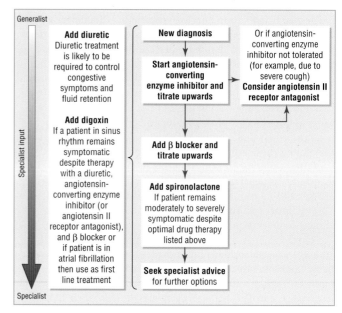

Algorithm for the pharmacological treatment of symptomatic heart failure caused by left ventricular systolic dysfunction. Adapted from National Institute for Health and Clinical Excellence clinical guideline 5: chronic heart failure: management of chronic heart failure in adults in primary and secondary care (www.nice.org.uk)

> Open access services have proved popular and are likely to become even more common; indeed, echocardiographic screening of patients in the high risk categories may well be justified and cost effective

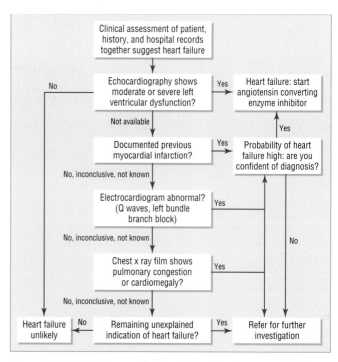

Diagnostic algorithm for suspected heart failure in primary care. Based on guidance from the north of England evidence based guideline development project

One approach may be to refer only those patients with abnormal results on baseline investigations as heart failure is unlikely if electrocardiography and chest x ray examination yield normal results and there are no predisposing factors for heart failure—for example, previous myocardial infarction, angina, hypertension, and diabetes mellitus. Requiring general practitioners to perform electrocardiography and arrange chest radiography, as a complement to careful assessment of the risk factors for heart failure, is likely to substantially reduce the number of inappropriate referrals to an open access echocardiography service.

Role of natriuretic peptides

Given the difficulties in diagnosing heart failure on clinical grounds alone, and current limited access to echocardiography and specialist assessment, the possibility of using a blood test in general practice to diagnose heart failure is appealing. Determining plasma concentrations of brain or B-type natriuretic peptide (BNP), a hormone found at an increased concentration in patients with left ventricular systolic dysfunction, may be one option. Such a blood test has the potential to screen out patients in whom heart failure is extremely unlikely and identify those in whom the probability of heart failure is high—for example, in patients with suspected heart failure who have low plasma concentrations of BNP, the heart is unlikely to be the cause of the symptoms, whereas those who have higher concentrations warrant further assessment.

Primary prevention and early detection

General practitioners have a vital role in the early detection and treatment of the main risk factors for heart failure—namely, hypertension and ischaemic heart disease—and other cardiovascular risk factors, such as smoking and hyperlipidaemia. The Framingham study has shown a decline in hypertension as a risk factor for heart failure over the years, which probably reflects improvements in treatment. Ischaemic heart disease, however, remains common. Aspirin, β blockers, and lipid lowering treatment, as well as smoking cessation, can reduce progression to myocardial infarction in patients with angina, and β blockers may also reduce ischaemic left ventricular dysfunction. Early detection of left ventricular dysfunction in "high risk" asymptomatic patients—for example, those who have already had a myocardial infarction or who have hypertension or atrial fibrillation—and treatment with ACE inhibitors can minimise the progression to symptomatic heart failure.

Starting and monitoring drug treatment

Both hospital doctors and general practitioners used to be concerned about the initiation of ACE inhibitors outside hospital. It is now accepted, however, that most patients with heart failure can safely be established on such treatment without needing hospital admission. The previous concern— over first dose hypotension—was heightened by the initial experience of large doses of captopril, especially in those with severe heart failure, who are at greater risk of problems. Patients with mild or moderate heart failure, who have normal renal function and a systolic blood pressure >100 mm Hg, rarely have problems, especially if the first dose of an ACE inhibitor is taken at bedtime.

Starting angiotensin converting enzyme (ACE) inhibitors in chronic heart failure in general practice
- Measure blood pressure and determine electrolytes and creatinine concentrations before treatment
- Consider referring "high risk" patients to hospital for assessment and supervised start of treatment
- ACE inhibitors should be used with some caution in patients with severe peripheral vascular disease because of the possible association with atherosclerotic renal artery stenosis
- Doses should be gradually increased over two to three weeks, aiming to reach the doses used in large clinical trials
- Perindopril and, to a lesser extent, ramipril require fewer dose titration steps than some other ACE inhibitors
- Blood pressure and electrolytes or renal chemistry should be monitored after start of treatment, initially at one week then less often depending on the patient and any abnormalities detected

> Recent studies have shown that with appropriate education of general practitioners the workload of an open access echocardiography service can be manageable

Conditions indicating that referral to a specialist is necessary
- Diagnosis in doubt or when specialist investigation and management may help
- Considerable murmurs and valvar heart disease
- Arrhythmias—for example, atrial fibrillation
- Secondary causes-for example, thyroid disease
- Severe left ventricular impairment—for example, ejection fraction <20%
- Pre-existing (or developing) metabolic abnormalities—for example, hyponatraemia (sodium <130 mmol/l) and renal impairment
- Severe associated vascular disease—caution with ACE inhibitors in case of coexisting renovascular disease
- Relative hypotension (systolic blood pressure <100 mm Hg before starting ACE inhibitors)
- Poor response to treatment

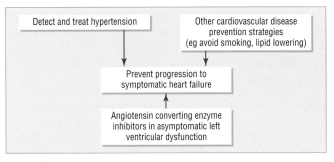

Strategies for preventing progression to symptomatic heart failure in high risk asymptomatic patients

Heart failure clinics

Dedicated heart failure clinics within general practices, run by a doctor or nurse with an interest in the subject, have the potential to improve the care of patients with the condition, as they have for other chronic conditions, such as diabetes.

Blood samples should be taken for electrolytes and renal chemistry at least every 12 months, and more often in new cases and when drug treatment has been changed or results have been abnormal. Blood lipid and sugar concentrations should also be checked at the same stage. The clinics should be used to educate patients about their condition, particularly in relation to their treatment, with messages being reinforced and drug treatment simplified and rationalised where appropriate. Patients whose condition is deteriorating may be referred for specialist opinion.

Variables that should be monitored in patients with established heart failure comprise changes in symptoms and severity (New York Heart Association classification), weight, blood pressure, and signs of fluid retention or excessive diuresis.

Impact of heart failure on the community

After a patient is diagnosed as having heart failure, substantial monitoring by the general practitioner is required. In our survey of heart failure in three general practices from the west of Birmingham, 44% of general practice consultations (average 2.6 visits per patient) took place within three months of the first diagnosis of heart failure, 23% were at three to six months (1.4 visits per patient), and 33% were at six to 12 months (2.0 visits per patient). Such management requires regular supervision and audit.

Relevance to hospital practice

In our survey of acute hospital admissions in patients with heart failure to a city centre hospital, the median duration of stay was eight (range 1–96) days, with 20% inpatient mortality. Clinical variables associated with an adverse prognosis include the presence of atrial fibrillation, poor exercise tolerance, electrolyte abnormalities, and the presence of coronary artery disease. ACE inhibitors were prescribed in only 51% of heart failure patients on discharge; after the first diagnosis of heart failure, the average number of hospital attendances (inpatient and outpatient) in the first 12 months was 3.2 visits per patient, with an average of 6.0 general practice consultations per patient. However, 44% of hospital attendances (1.4 visits per patient) took place within three months of diagnosis, 33% were at three to six months (1.0 visits per patient), and 23% were at 6–12 months (0.74 visits per patient).

These figures represent the collective burden of heart failure on hospital practice. Indeed, about 200 000 people in the UK require admission to hospital for heart failure each year.

General practitioners with special interest

With an ageing population and fewer junior doctors being available to see patients in hospital outpatient clinics because of changes in working hours, along with patients' preference to be managed in the community, general practitioners with special

Assessments to be made at clinical review

Assessment	
Functional capacity	Chiefly from history, but more objectively by use of NYHA class, specific questionnaires on quality of life, a six minute walk test, or maximal exercise test. Note: not all of these tests will be necessary, or appropriate, at each assessment
Fluid status	Chiefly by physical examination—changes in body weight, extent of jugular venous distension, lung crackles, and hepatomegaly; extent of peripheral oedema; and lying and standing blood pressure (postural drop in pressure may indicate hypovolaemia)
Cardiac rhythm	Chiefly by clinical examination but may require 12 lead electrocardiogram or 24 hour electrocardiographic (Holter) monitoring if suspicion of arrhythmia
Laboratory	Checking of serum biochemistry (urea, electrolytes, creatine) is essential, but other tests (such as thyroid function, haematology, liver function, level of anticoagulation) may also be required depending on the medication prescribed and comorbidity

Adapted from National Institute for Health and Clinical Excellence clinical guideline 5: chronic heart failure: management of chronic heart failure in adults in primary and secondary care (www.nice.org.uk)

Causes of readmission in patients with heart failure

- Angina
- Infections
- Arrhythmias
- Poor compliance
- Inadequate drug treatment
- Iatrogenic factors
- Inadequate discharge planning or follow-up
- Poor social support

Examples of topics for audit for heart failure management in general practice

Means of diagnosis
- Has left ventricular function been assessed by echocardiography or other means?

Appropriateness of treatment
- Are all appropriate patients taking ACE inhibitors (unless there is a documented contraindication)?
- Have doses been increased when possible to those used in the large clinical trials?

Monitoring treatment
- Were blood pressure and renal function recorded before and after the start of ACE inhibitors and at intervals subsequently?

interest (GPSIs) are increasingly conducting clinics in their own surgeries, seeing not only their own patients but those of their colleagues, both from their own practice and in some cases neighbouring ones. Large, multi-partner practices with suitable accommodation available for such clinics have facilitated their introduction, and the new general practitioner contract in England and Wales has also provided an impetus, as practices receive payments if quality standards are documented as having been met.

Heart failure is in many ways an ideal condition for such general practitioners to be involved in as patients are often elderly and poorly mobile and would therefore prefer to see a doctor with an interest in their condition near to home. It may be possible to see patients more often in a community clinic because of lack of availability of appointments in hospitals, and, as medication can be directly prescribed by the GPSI rather than recommendations being given by hospital doctors, which may not be followed, patients are more likely to receive full dose, evidence based medications.

As well as follow-up, GPSIs may play an important part in the diagnosis of heart failure. With portable echocardiography now being possible in the community, comprehensive assessment of patients no longer requires visits to hospital, and community diagnostic clinics have been successfully instituted in some areas. In addition to studying those with suspected heart failure, practice records can be examined for those with risk factors for heart failure (especially ischaemic heart disease and diabetes) and those who have not undergone echocardiography could be called up for a study in their own practice. Our research showed that 22% of those with a record of myocardial infarction in their general practice notes had a left ventricular ejection fraction <40%, with borderline left ventricular function (ejection fraction 40–50%) in a further 20%. Thus the yield from screening such patients is likely to be high.

Quality control, especially for echocardiography, is important when practitioners are working autonomously in the community. Good links with local cardiologists are essential for a good GPSI service. A diploma course has recently been instituted at the University of Bradford for GPSIs in cardiology, and similar courses are being set up elsewhere.

Economic considerations

With an increasingly elderly population, the prevalence of heart failure is likely to continue to increase in the coming years, with attendant costs. Some interventions—for example, ACE inhibitors and β blockers, now available generically—and specialist nursing services are likely to be cost neutral or even save money because of the associated reduction in hospital admissions. Other interventions—for example, prophylactic implantable cardioverter defibrillators—are extremely expensive and may not be a cost effective use of resources in some healthcare systems.

In 2000 the direct cost of heart failure to the NHS in the UK was estimated at £905m, or nearly 1.91% of total NHS expenditure. Admissions to hospital accounted for 69% of this and drug prescriptions 18%. Indirect costs (secondary admissions and nursing home care for those with heart failure) account for a further equivalent of 2%. Admissions for heart failure have been increasing and are expected to increase further. Preventing disease progression, hence reducing the frequency and duration of admissions, is therefore an important objective both in terms of patients' quality of life and also in economic terms in the treatment of heart failure in the future.

> Heart failure is likely to continue to become a major public health problem in the coming decades; new and better management strategies are necessary, including risk factor interventions, for patients at risk of developing heart failure

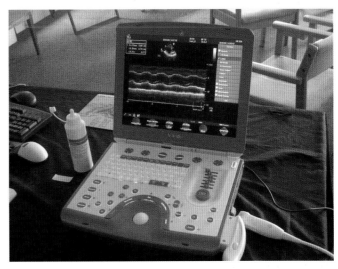

High quality echocardiography equipment is now portable

Further reading

- Davis RC, Hobbs FDR, Kenkre JE, Roalfe AK, Hare R. Prevalence of left ventricular systolic dysfunction and heart failure in high risk patients: community based epidemiological study. *BMJ* 2002;1156–8.
- Francis CM, Caruana L, Kearney P, Love M, Sutherland GR, Starkey IR, et al. Open access echocardiography in the management of heart failure in the community. *BMJ* 1995;310:634–6.
- Remes J, Miettinen H, Reunanen A, Pyorala K. Validity of clinical diagnosis of heart failure in primary health care. *Eur Heart J* 1991;12:315–21.
- Rich MW, Beckham V, Wittenberg C, Leven CL, Freedland KE, Carney RM, et al. A multidisciplinary intervention to prevent the readmission of elderly patients with congestive heart failure. *N Engl J Med* 1995;333:1190–5.
- Stewart S, Jenkins A, Buchan S, McGuire A, Capewell S, McMurray JJV. The current cost of heart failure to the National Health Service in the UK. *Eur J Heart Fail* 2002;4:361–71
- Stewart S, Vandenbroek AJ, Pearson S, Horowitz JD. Prolonged beneficial effects of home-based intervention on unplanned readmissions and mortality among patients with congestive heart failure. *Arch Intern Med* 1999;159:257–61.

This chapter was adapted from the corresponding one in the first edition written by FDR Hobbs, RC Davis, and GYH Lip. Our colleague's previous contribution is gratefully acknowledged.

Index

Index

Index

leg ulceration 50
lethargy 15
levosimendan 43
LIDO study 43
lifestyle measures 25–7, 44
limb ischaemia 50
lipid lowering treatment 55
lisinopril 19, 35
liver function 22
losartan 36
low output heart failure 16
lung disease 17
lung function 24
lungs, bat's wing appearance 22

MADIT-II study 30, 31
magnesium levels 22
magnetic resonance imaging (MRI) 24
  gadolinium enhancement 23, 45
malnutrition 27
medication *see* drug therapy
MERIT-HF study 38
metabolic acidosis 42
metolazone 34, 45
metoprolol 38, 39
milrinone 40
mitral incompetence 21, 45
mitral regurgitation 7, 8, 45
MONICA study 2, 3
morphine 42
mortality 18
  angiotensin receptor antagonists 36
  congestive heart failure 30
  defibrillator implantation 30, 31
  digoxin 39
  exercise training impact 27–8
  ischaemic heart disease 30
  maternal in left ventricular dysfunction 26
  natriuretic peptide predictors 23
  QRS complex width 29
  resynchronisation therapy 30
  resynchronisation/defibrillatory combined therapy 31–2
  specialist nursing services 47, 49, 51
myocardial infarction 6
  angiotensin receptor antagonists 36
  atrial fibrillation 17
  digoxin contraindication 39
  displaced apex beat 16
  myocardial remodelling 10, 13
  progression prevention 55
  risk for heart failure 55
  ventricular tachycardia 17
myocardial ischaemia 21
myocarditis, viral 6, 8
myocardium
  biopsy 7, 23
  fibrosis 7
  hibernating 14, 24, 28, 45
  impaired relaxation 52
  remodelling 10, 13, 14
  systolic dysfunction 10
myxoedema 9

natriuretic peptides 10, 11–12, 22–3
  determination in general practice 55
nebivolol 38
nephron, diuretic action 33, 34
nesiritide 43
neurohormonal activation 10–12, 12
neutral endopeptidase 12
New York Heart Association (NYHA) classification 16, 18
nitrates, oral 36–7, 43

nitric oxide 13
non-invasive positive pressure ventilation (NPPV) 43
non-steroidal anti-inflammatory drugs (NSAIDs),
    contraindication 42
norepinephrine (noradrenaline) 11, 12, 35
N-terminal pro-brain natriuretic peptide (NT-proBNP) 12,
    22–3
nurses, specialist 47–51, 57
nursing services, clinical effectiveness 51
nutrition 27, 50

obesity 27
oedema 15
  congestive heart failure 34
  see also pulmonary oedema
opiates/opioids 42, 50
orthopnoea 15
oxygen, smoking effects 26
oxygen delivery 42

pacing, biventricular 29
pain management 50
palliative care 49–50
paroxysmal nocturnal dyspnoea 15
pathophysiology of heart failure 10–14
patients
  deterioration detection 48–9
  medication titration 48
  see also education of patients
peak expiratory flow rate 24
PEP-CHF study 53
pericardial disease 5
perindopril 53
pharmaceuticals *see* drug therapy
pharmacists 49
phosphodiesterase inhibitors 43
physical deconditioning 27
physical signs 15–16
polyarteritis nodosa 6
polypharmacy 47–8
positron emission tomography (PET) 45
potassium levels 22, 34, 45
  supplementation 22, 33
PRAISE study 37
pre-menopausal women, dilated cardiomyopathy 26
pressure area care 50
prevalence of heart disease 2–3, 57
primary care *see* general practice
primary prevention 55
PRIME II trial 40
prognosis 18–19
  adverse 56
prolonged QT interval 17
proteinuria 22
PROVED trial 39
pulmonary embolism 17, 19
pulmonary function tests 24
pulmonary oedema 22, 42, 43
pulmonary venous congestion 22

QRS complex, width 29

RADIANCE study 39
radionuclide studies 24, 45
RALES study 34
red blood cells, technetium-99m labelled 24
relatives, counselling/education 25, 44, 47
renal artery stenosis 21–2
renal function 21–2
renin–angiotensin–aldosterone system (RAAS) 10–11, 13
respiratory infections 8
respite care 50